FROM
PAIN TO
POSSIBILITY

FROM PAIN TO POSSIBILITY

Remember your way home
to the true and advanced you!

Mark Worthington

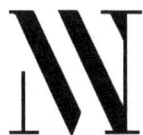

First published 2024 by Mark Worthington.

www.mark-worthington.com

Copyright © Mark Worthington 2024

The moral rights of the author have been asserted.

All rights reserved. No part of this book may be reproduced or transmitted by any person or entity, including internet search engines or retailers (including, but not restricted to, Google and Amazon), in any form or by any means, electronic or mechanical, including photocopying (except under the statutory exceptions provisions of the Australian Copyright Act 1968), recording, scanning or by any information storage and retrieval system without the prior written permission of the author.

The author expressly prohibits any entity from using this publication in any manner for purposes of training artificial intelligence (AI) technologies to generate text, including without limitation technologies that are capable of generating works in the same style or genre as this publication. The author reserves all rights to license uses of this work for generative AI training and development of machine learning language models.

Because of the dynamic nature of the internet, any web addresses or links contained in this book may have changed since publication and may no longer be valid. The author of this book does not dispense medical advice or prescribe the use of any technique as a form of treatment for physical, emotional, or medical problems without the advice of a physician, either directly or indirectly. The intent of the author is only to offer information of a general nature to help you in your quest for emotional and spiritual wellbeing. In the event you use any of the information in this book for yourself, which is your constitutional right, the author assumes no responsibility for your actions.

Cover design by Julia Kuris, Designerbility designerbility.com.au

Internal design by Zena Shapter, zenashapter.com

Diagrams and Pictures by Bill Shapter, posbycheckout.com

CONTENTS

INTRODUCTION   9
   Are You Ready to Embrace Advanced Normality?   9

WE ARE ALL METAPHYSICAL   27
   Chapter 1: Core Metaphysical Concepts   28
   Chapter 2: Controls Over Our Fate   42
   Chapter 3: The Vibrational Power of Nature   50
   Chapter 4: Our Vibrational Connectivity   55
   Chapter 5: Your Way, Your Truth, Your Light   66

WE CHOOSE OUR OWN PATH   83
   Chapter 6: The Choices We Must Make   84
   Chapter 7: My Path Through Pain to Infinite Possibilities   90
   Chapter 8: Preparing For Your Enlightenment   98
   Chapter 9: The Battle Between Ego and Soul Energy   113

PAIN IS INEVITABLE   **121**
   Chapter 10: How Pain is Misunderstood   122

HOW TO MAKE USE OF PAIN   **129**
   Chapter 11: The Normal Way We Deal With Pain   130
   Chapter 12: The Natural Arc of Human Transformation   144
   Chapter 13: A Case Study of Unlearning   174
   Chapter 14: Overcoming Physical Pain   188
   Chapter 15: Ownership of Pain   203

Chapter 16: Losing the Plot in Our Pain	210
Chapter 17: The Love You Truly Seek	220
Chapter 18: You Will Not Be Alone	227

THE POSSIBILITIES AWAITING YOU — 231

Chapter 19: Manifesting Beyond the Mind	232
Chapter 20: What Becomes Possible	237
Chapter 21: Receiving Intelligences	250
Chapter 22: Living in the Energies of Gratitude and Trust	254
Chapter 23: Advanced Self-Awareness Experiences	259

RETURNING HOME — 279

Chapter 24: Remembering What You Already Are	280

CONCLUDING REMARKS — 287

Chapter 25: The Mystical Quest	288

Acknowledgements — 295

About the Author — 297

This book is primarily dedicated to love.

Love has been the source of all knowing in my life and is therefore the architect of the wonderful journey I have taken to know myself. By allowing love to own me and overwhelm me, rather than the other way around, I have learned and unlearned my way into now living a beautiful and happy life.

Truth is also a powerful energy that has ignited and extinguished all the key phases of my life and led me to discover new possibilities. I will never live without truth again, for to do so would be too painful to endure.

I also dedicate this book to pain, for ultimately my pain was a significant source of inspiration that steered me to new possibilities and fresh beginnings. Recognising the loving messages that my pain had for me, allowed me to evolve to a place where pain is now only a fleeting, but valuable experience, in my life.

Finally, I am grateful that the spirit realm has graced my life with many wonderful metaphysical experiences and understandings over the last nine years. These unsolicited happenings have shown me the clarity of my own reality, and allowed me to now share this reality with my readers, not to 'big note' myself, but to support my version of the truth for others to consider.

Mark Worthington
Author

INTRODUCTION

Are You Ready to Embrace Advanced Normality?

This book is a summary of what I learnt over nine years on my journey to higher conscious awareness, and through seven years of responding to coaching from metaphysical mentors. It is raw and true, and for the first time introduces the metaphysical into my work on consciousness in a big way.

Consciousness is largely metaphysical, and most of humanity has lost its memory of what can be allowed to grace their lives when people truly align themselves with the wisdom of their souls. We are largely unaware of what is possible when we find the way home to our true selves.

Let me say this upfront: you are here to remember the truth of yourself and to discover the true experience of being yourself. This is the ultimate adventure for a human being – to become completely conscious while in human form.

Meditation and spiritual modalities do help and are an important entry point into the consciousness journey, but it only provides a moderate incursion into the totality of our individual truths. How do I know this? I did it too in the early stages of my awakening!

So, if you sense that there is more to life than you have been taught or currently understand, then you are an evolved reader with an enquiring mind, and this book is probably for you.

Anyone who is curious enough to want to discover their true capabilities and greatest happiness can take the paths outlined in these pages. We are entering a time in the Earth's evolution when, collectively, we have the energetic support from the universe to remember what we truly are, and to find higher consciousness awareness.

By following the model that I put forward in this book, anyone can start down the path to become fully connected to their soul 24/7, and experience all that that entails. I have walked this path now for over nine years, with high-powered mentors guiding me, so I know what is possible.

As you read this book, you will find that my personal experiences, as I walked my own path, are highlighted in bold italic text. These are all true experiences. I appreciate some readers may not seek to venture into these, for they are merely my experiences, and theirs may be very different. Still, I share them to give readers a reference point and examples they can choose to consider, if this is their preference.

I have been gifted with many amazing metaphysical experiences and I share some of these in this book. I do not take these for granted, nor do I consider them to be any kind of achievement that could be seen to make me seem more important in any way. I hope readers do not perceive this kind of ego-centric outcome to be my intent. I'm just an ordinary person who has had some interesting experiences, which may assist others if they are shared.

I am merely fortunate that they were bestowed upon me by the universe to assist me, in divine timing, with my own awakening process. All of these events occurred 'out of the blue' and were unsolicited. I know that my mind is not capable of planning or creating these types of experiences – but my soul is, as is yours.

I thus share them with readers to provide a sense of the kind of experiences that can take place when we are ready to encounter and participate in new paradigms, without the barriers installed by our own fear.

What matters is often not matter; experiences like the ones I describe in this book can serve to challenge our preconceived understandings of life. They certainly did that for me.

Pain and Joy Are Messages of Love

Pain is a source of wisdom that we have come to hate, a message of love from the soul that we too often choose to ignore and suppress. While we welcome feelings of joy when it graces our lives, both joy *and* pain arise within us from the same source.

The model I put forward in this book can assist you in arising from pain as a source of unhappiness and allow you to rediscover happiness through pain. It may not readily apply to pain that is completely and utterly beyond your personal control, and to which you are not directly contributing, such as pain derived from accidents, conflicts, or diseases. Although a person may have somehow contributed to its existence, medical intervention may be the most potent assistance a sufferer possesses in such instances.

But if you have any emotional or psychological pain, if you are experiencing any physical manifestations of that emotional or psychological pain, if you have any pain that you have contributed to through your beliefs, energies, or mindsets, then my model can help you to discover extraordinary levels of joy and to embark on new beginnings.

I have healed myself both emotionally and physically by loving and respecting my pain using my model. By simply learning from my pain and changing my beliefs I was able to end my physical and emotional suffering. I consciously chose this outcome.

This book has the potential to redefine how mankind looks at certain kinds of pain altogether, including stress and depression. But more importantly it may improve the way you experience your own life!

After many years of suffering from great stress and grief in my life, I eventually realised that the various experiences of pain I felt inside my body were warnings that I was in some way out of step with my true self, and that I would be well served to consider different ways of living my life. The pain was prompting me to reassess my previous choices, and it would not go away easily, such was the depths of its love for me.

I had to really love my pain, for my pain really loved me. It was a gift that took me far too long to unwrap. It was a friend that I once saw as my enemy.

Learning to grow from both pain and joy is an important part of the human condition and the universal experiment in which we are invited to participate. Life is a journey of discovery, an opportunity to experience love and learning, and the clearest discoveries arise through our feelings and how we interpret them.

We are like a great ocean. The waves upon its surface, and the changing colours that appear as the weather impacts upon it, are akin to the many experiences and emotions that we so often go through. But the truth of the ocean lies within its depths; its external features are but temporary. We need to look within ourselves in order to experience life at its fullest, and that involves appreciating both joy and pain.

Highs and lows allow our conscious awareness to expand, affording us the opportunity to replace fear with love. We may all want a life without lows, this is normal; but it is not natural, and to expect this anomaly sets us up for disappointments and periods of 'perceived' failure. Witnessing life as the roller-coaster that it can be, allows us to be free of the inherent need we so often develop to always succeed, and be seen as perfect in the eyes of ourselves and others, as we are all conditioned to do.

But if we can sense into the possibilities that await us, when we practice letting our preconceived views of life go, we can give ourselves a great gift. It may not alter our current circumstances in a hurry, but it can change the way we feel about them.

True happiness, derived from the inner knowing of yourself is critical to remembering the happiness you are capable of embodying. Why not centre your true source of light and ignite your true radiance? This can lead you to new horizons and a new ocean of dreams.

Throwing yourself at the waves of life, with a desire to grow and expand, is the constant refreshment that your heart wants you to have. The key is to truly surrender to the journey of self-discovery that your life force brings forth into your awareness.

Key Propositions to Ponder

To apply the concepts in this book, it helps if you can accept the proposition that we are eternal beings, and that this life is not an isolated event. Life has a complex interrelationship with the evolutionary experiences we will experience as we journey through lifetime after lifetime. We are all metaphysical.

The next step is to appreciate that people don't just carry emotional pain from this life, but in the form of karma from past lives. Karma sometimes means that a certain experience must be had in this life to balance past wrongdoings. The 'university of life' on this planet can be unpleasant at times. That's why learning from your experiences and pain is so important – it can stop them from repeating in your universal thread, including the rest of your current life. In this wisdom, we choose our own path to happiness.

Many people struggle to believe in the concept of a loving universe on the basis that they observe bad things happening in the world and to themselves. This is an understandable viewpoint; but it is born out of ignorance as to how universal energies work. We all came here to live from love and expand, and that expansion is normally derived from learning through suffering. It doesn't have to be that way, but the reality is that we tend to learn less from positive experiences. Therefore, pain is largely inevitable and very hard to avoid in our lives.

In unlearning what and who we think we are, however, we can open up a gateway to tempering or removing a great deal of our pain altogether, and allow our true selves to burst forth through us. Pain – especially psychological and emotional pain – can be a fleeting experience once we learn to love it and learn from it. My model shows you how to make use of pain, and to grow through it.

Opening to our pain allows us to shed light on what density and beliefs are blocking us from merging with the full consciousness that is alive within our hearts.

Are You Really Ready?

Be warned, this book is not for everyone. It contains very advanced principles on what is possible when you take the inner journey to find your true self. This book is only for those among us who want to and are ready to embrace an advanced normality, and find out who they were truly meant to be. This may require you to drop the story of who you currently think you are, and open to a more natural reality.

At present, humanity fears many of the truths I have learned from the metaphysical realms within which we exist, and that fear holds us back from co-creating with the universe and discovering our true capabilities. Many believe that we are separate from God and each other, and this is the source of great personal suffering. It makes us unlovable, if we fail. But we are not meant to live in this separation consciousness. We are truly all one and not alone in this world.

My book doesn't just put forward advanced spiritual principles, it contains a practical model that anyone can use to attain greater consciousness and embrace their full 'power to love' on Earth. This power is derived from connecting to our truths and does not conform with the normal principles of power with which most of us are familiar. Power over another is not true power. Love is the real source of power, and unlimited possibilities await you when you open to your divine self.

Those who are fully connected to their souls and their light can access what we typically call 'psychic powers' beyond their wildest dreams, for they can access more of the super-powers of their metaphysical selves. These are discussed in more detail in this book.

A truly wonderful experience that anyone on Earth can have is to unleash and embrace their full divinity while living in this 3D world, and to apply this to the physical realm. That's why this book is only for the advanced among us who can accept the duality of our own reality, and who want to explore how far they can truly expand, become and create.

We are all spirits living a physical existence and opening to this truth is the only way to experience higher conscious awareness and transcend the more rudimentary security consciousness most people have been taught to accept.

The Bliss That Awaits

As we increase our conscious awareness, we can't help but get lighter in every respect, even physically. When we embrace the truth, the illusions and limiting beliefs that we once let define the way we feel and live, we are brought out of the shadows and into the light, and we can let love, not fear, guide us forward.

In this magical place, all aspects of our being can become more radiant, and we can experience more fun and love. Who does not want that?

Higher conscious awareness will show you where you are being too serious in life, and in turn diminishing the happiness you are here on this planet to experience.

My model can't promise you that you will find your super-powers, or even have the full experience of finding your true self, that's between you and God, but I'm confident that it will allow you to choose a happier experience of your life.

Our ego-centric minds can be great assets in our lives, but they can also be the source of much pain. Purifying our conditioned beliefs and thoughts is the only true and sustainable way to happiness. All other strategies are temporary, at best, for the human ego can rarely be fully satisfied, and in moments of disruption it will lead us to despair, unless our sense of self is real and not based on the illusions of conditioned thinking and external validation.

My book *Where Your Happiness Hides* defined the path to individual *happiness* by offering readers a code of happiness that could lead them to a better world. It also showed readers how their belief structures largely determine the quality of their lives and why they essentially become conditioned and unhappy. My book *Show Me The Harmony* showed readers how *harmony* can be attained in collectives and how authentic leadership can help to create this.

I was drawn to write these books because, when we are all happy within ourselves and accept our own uniqueness, we can come together in a united and harmonious way that can create a better world for everyone. Life is not about fitting in and competing from a place of conformity. Higher consciousness is the key to breaking this distorted nexus.

Both of these books were intentionally and partially silent on the power of the metaphysical in our lives. Metaphysical concepts are not accepted by everyone, but few are averse to considering the existence of our beliefs and their impact on our lives.

Mainstream thinking is typically resistant to accepting the concepts and realities that spirituality brings forth, mostly out of conditioned fear, although this is gradually changing. What we are wrongly taught in western cultures is that: matter is all that truly matters. This book goes to a higher level of truth in this regard.

Time to Return Home?

It is now possible for everyone, with this book, to choose to return home to their full truths and allow the complete bliss that lives within them to arise through them and for them. Universal energies and your spirit realm are now fully in support of this opportunity becoming possible for us all.

But first you need to be aware of it, and then to want it. This book provides this awareness to the open-hearted reader, and the well-known quest for the holy grail becomes a metaphor in this, for finding your true self. The holy grail can only be found by truly knowing thyself. Know yourself and you can eliminate much of the suffering you may be enduring in your mind and body every day.

The universe is ever expanding, as are we, for we are all an important part of the universe. We are here to learn this, should we choose to; for life happens *for* us and *through* us – it never happens *to* us, though this is what many have come to believe. Taking full responsibility for your life is a foreign concept in many cultures, yet it is the only way that we can discover our true and natural selves, before finding our own way home.

I have therefore used my own experiences to develop a natural process of transformation, from which others can easily learn, called the Natural Arc of Human Transformation (the Arc).

This book advances a reader's understanding of how the three core aspects of our beings – our minds, bodies, and spirits – can naturally interact to transform the actual experiences of our lives, and how by understanding these relationships we can react and respond to issues of mental and physical health, including pain, in a more natural and conscious way. The process has turned my life from one of confusion into one of great clarity, so I know just how effectively the Arc works.

Even though I was a highly educated individual, I truly had no idea who and what I really was until I explored the concepts of consciousness outlined in this book, deeply and with integrity. So let me now share my journey with you, so you can discover your true self, hopefully without the misadventures I encountered!

We all talk about doing creative things and being creative. But the fact is that you *are* the creator, and we are all here to connect to our full source of creativity. Creation is intrinsically what you are!

You are the pure energy of love. This is your natural way of being and has been with you for eternity. It always will be. These energies can never be permanently turned off, and they are yours to access should you choose to do the work needed to bring them forth.

The truth of you, once you discover it, will blow the primitive apparatus that currently thinks it is the real you – your mind – and relegate it to its more natural role, as a support act.

The real you can give you access to a state of happiness and joy, and powers, beyond your wildest dreams. Becoming advanced normality awaits your attention. Are you ready for that experience?

Natural Advancement Is Not For Everyone – Yet!

We are all at different stages of our evolution to higher consciousness. We are all on different paths, and we all have different intentions in living our respective lives.

Some people are just here to enjoy life and are content to experience, what could be termed more normal things, like having a family, having a good career or falling in love. Their lives are all they want them to be, and they see no need to change. That is just where they are at on their path, and that is a completely valid choice. Others are here to expand and grow beyond the current paradigms within which they live. We are all equal, no matter what we choose. Having a high enough consciousness to choose what we want with wisdom is the key.

However, if you do not understand what is truly possible in your life how can you ever make a fully informed choice? You cannot!

As the universal energies, which I mentioned above, shift to higher frequencies, many may suffer more than they have become accustomed to, if they are living from the fear in their egos and not the love in their hearts. This may cause them confusion and pain. As human beings we are unlikely to embrace transformation unless we have been challenged by loss. This is our normal way of living.

Evolution allows for everything to unfold as intended, but we can co-create and assist with our evolution if we embrace the opportunity to do so in a willing way, and work with our souls.

Our respective energetic diversities are just timing differences, in a universe that truly disregards time. Being a normal human being is often challenging and complex. Suffering and pain are as common as happiness and joy, unfortunately; and for some they see no other way than to simply endure those many highs and lows.

This was once my paradigm of life, until I saw the light.

We are also very capable beings, and some of us, as I alluded to above, are here because we want to expand to a higher place of evolution, find our way back to our eternal truth, and discover what we are truly capable of by developing deep self-connection. Your 'gut' will tell you which of these types of people you are at present. Your intuition will tell you if you want normality, or if you are ready for the more advanced experiences that are possible. All you need to do is listen to its messages and discern what you want your path to include.

At some point, your desire to understand your divine purpose may be sparked into action and tempt you to expand your consciousness. However, you must be energetically ready for this to be brought forth into this 3D reality. This is often referred to as an awakening.

The wisdom encoded and embodied in this book allows for your activation to be possible in this life, but only should you choose it. I say *encoded*, for this book has been written with the assistance of higher intelligence infused from beyond our 3D world, and its conditioned ways of thinking. Much of it has been channelled through me and is written for your heart and not just your mind.

However, if you do not feel ready to journey to advanced consciousness just yet, then give this book to someone who is ready *now*. Your time will come eventually, at some point in your evolutionary thread, because evolution is inherently unstoppable. It's okay, however, if this is not the right time for you to take this journey.

Understanding Our Shifting World

If you are ready to take this journey, you should be encouraged, because spiritual concepts are gracing our world more and more each day, as people awaken and begin to question their lives. Many of the principles brought forth in this book are at the cutting-edge of what might be referred to as spirituality. But they are also important when you understand what is happening for our planet and beyond, and therefore for you. Allow me to share the following awarenesses with you.

All is energy. Living in this world is, therefore, an energetic experience. The Earth has been energetically dense for centuries. However, we are amid a major energetic shift for the Earth and the galaxy of which we are a part. The frequencies or vibrations we are living within are lifting at the will of God and are taking us into a different experience. This vibration represents a new dimensional blending of frequencies that is taking us closer to the vibration of universal love.

This is a great positive for our world, but it comes with great challenges, and for some great pain will arise as we transition. Transformation is change on steroids, and we are currently on the precipice of this great shift. These higher energies, sometimes referred to as being the vibration of the New Earth, are exaggerating the energies of fear and love that we all hold, and are in turn impacting on our experiences.

You cannot be in this experience of higher energies and have the same experiences of yourself in the third dimension that we inhabit, if you are clinging to old, conditioned ideas of yourself. This frequency will demand that you evolve with it, and the only way to do so is through your soul, or true self.

The energy within your soul knows your future and your divine purpose or meaning of your life. It is encoded with a divinity code that will be activated once you are deemed ready for it to do so. Your ego is unaware of your divine intentions and cannot activate this divinity.

So, who do you think it's best to trust with your future: the personality or fake identity of yourself that was derived in the past, or your true self that knows your intended future and why you are here now to experience this energetic transformation in which you and the world exist? Can you trust your ego to take you into a future that it does not understand, and cannot know, until it becomes the past?

To enjoy a positive experience of this transformative period, your ego must surrender to the life force within you, which has the encoded frequencies that are being activated inside you now. To do otherwise is likely to bring you great pain and distress. This book attempts to bring you the awareness, so that you may transform with this energetic shift with as little effort and suffering as possible.

How do I know this? Because I have already been through much suffering at the hands of my own ego in this dimensional shift and have had the opportunity to discuss it with higher powers.

You will not become your embodied, divine self if you do not bring your awareness to your truth in your soul. The model in this book allows that to commence, so that your soul can show you your truth and take you into the vibration of true love.

Only the God-essence within you has the power to take you to pure consciousness, but you can bring your density and distorted beliefs into the light by using my model, so that your divinity can burst forth into your life at the right moment.

The enlightenment or awakening process that this book outlines, is one that many of us will naturally seek to pursue at some stage in our lives. Often it is triggered by losses or disruptions in our lives that make us question what our life is all about, and why such losses have occurred. We seek to make sense of our existence and what has taken place for us.

Armed with the wisdom that others have probably already discovered, many of us set off on a spiritual path. This can start us on a journey of revelation. But, unless we understand how it can unfold, it can also cause us great disappointment and even delusions, as we fail to meet our expectations.

We typically approach our awakening through our egos and conditioned ways of being, treating it like a project or task we need to complete. Using our methodical minds to orchestrate our unfolding is helpful, but there comes a point at which we must fully surrender to our true source of consciousness. Our minds will think that they are our source of pure consciousness, but this is a falsehood.

As you take part in spiritual modalities or other sources of new awareness, seeking to be the enlightened one, you will eventually discover that all your hard work and trying can never get you to the point you dream about. All your work is helpful because it reveals or sheds light on the beliefs that you need to release to rediscover or remember what you really are. Eventually you see that the soul within you is already complete and is the very outcome that you seek. The barrier to its full presence is you.

For most, the advanced step into their light is one of complete surrender, of accepting and trusting where you are, and allowing yourself to be immersed in the life force that you ultimately are. To make this final step into the light you must be aligned with the vibration of love. Light can only spring forth from the frequency of universal love.

Along the journey to enlightenment, your mind is both your enemy and your friend. However, it can never, ever take you to your full conscious awareness, because it has no concept of what that is or entails. It is temporary apparatus that only exists in this life.

You are a fountain of life force able to overflow into the world and to step into your fullness. However, to do this you must give up believing that you know who and what you really are. Your mind has no idea of this truth, only your soul has that divine knowing. And the greatest challenge for any human being is to give up the identity or personality that they spent a lifetime creating, and allow love to show you who and what you chose to be before you arrived on this planet.

We come to Earth and create new plans and senses of purpose, unaware that we have already chosen our intended path with the divine will of God before we are born.

Knowing thyself is a wonderful outcome of trusting yourself and accepting that your truth is beyond your current consciousness. Only the consciousness that is possible in your soul and the will of God can bring it to your attention.

As is often said, to solve a problem we are best placed to do so from a higher level of consciousness to the one that created the issue in the first place. Your soul gives you unlimited consciousness that is far beyond that of the mind, if you choose to discover it. With access to this divine knowing, you have powers and abilities beyond your comprehension to make this life far more successful and easier for you. Once you know, your life will flow.

I would recommend that you open to this truth, for to stay 'stuck' in traditional and conditioned ways of thinking, is likely to lead you into pain, if it hasn't already.

Find Your Flow

Evolution is like a river, flowing from the mountains to the sea. It will sometimes stagnate, awaiting a new burst of energy in the form of rain, to allow it to flow to a new terrain, but ultimately its waters will make the journey that they must, to the great oceans, where they will be unconditionally welcomed as an important part of the whole. From here, the water will evaporate into clouds, only to return to the lands as new sources of life and energy, making the journey back to the river as individual droplets of rain. Such is the path of our own realities as we reincarnate lifetime after lifetime.

The only question for you right now is: how do you want your journey to the sea to be like in this incarnation? Do you want to be the energy that makes a great river flow as a powerful rapid, or do you want to float more slowly through more stagnate waters in a less challenging way? Do you want to make it in full authenticity to the great ocean in this life, because you chose to discover and embrace the true you? Are you feeling the energetic shifts in the river and can you feel a desire to go with this flow to avoid the difficulties of crossing the current?

But you have to choose it with your heart. You must feel it; you cannot think it. If you attempt to just think it, you are likely to limit your journey to the safe option that you already understand, or take it on because of an egoic desire to win, presuming that being advanced makes you better than others. Let me be clear, it does not!

But your journey is not part of a competition with any prize at the end, other than your own sense of authenticity and happiness. So, comparisons to the consciousness levels of others are neither advisable, nor truly possible, if you choose to open to the truth, because regardless of our relative consciousness levels we are all equal forever.

When I was unexpectantly offered the opportunity to follow a path to higher consciousness, by higher beings that graced my path, I accepted that opportunity without a moment's hesitation. I just knew and felt it was for me. You will know whether it's for you, one way or another. This book speaks to the open-hearted and open-minded and gives them truths that they can use to make their own life choices. I desire nothing more.

The Wonder of Challenge

The path to higher consciousness can challenge all that you think you know of yourself. It will change you, though you won't know to what extent until it unfolds in grace. Only your soul will know the answer to that question, and it will only share it with your mind when you are truly ready to hear it.

Like anything worthwhile in life, this path requires commitment and diligence. It is not an easy road to take, depending on your circumstances, and it may seem overwhelming and lonely at times.

I have been down this difficult and sometimes lonely road, but I accepted every pothole and speed bump with the greatest grace I could muster.

You will need to stare deeply into your realities and have the personal integrity to pull yourself apart and put yourself back together, piece by piece. At times, it will be like standing naked in front of a mirror, because you will be installed as the witness of your perceived imperfections. As your self-compassion grows, you will eventually see the reflection of your true inner and outer beauty and know that you are perfect in your imperfections. The truth of you will be witnessed in the light in your eyes, for your eyes are truly the window to your soul, as is so often said.

Personally, I cannot imagine a greater gift you could give yourself, than getting to know the real and wonderful you. What could be more worthwhile than making the journey to know yourself, and the loving gifts you can bring to this great planet, both for yourself and for others?

But whether you are ready or not, whether you are normal or advanced normal, you will always remain wonderful, and an irreplaceable part of the loving tapestry of this universe.

We are all unique, and I marvel at the incredible traits and wonders of everyone with whom I come into contact and connect. We are all natural wonders of this world, and truly amazing – there are no exceptions to this!

Since this book takes you on the journey I encountered along my path to higher consciousness, its chapters and sections are structured so that they mirror what I encountered, and what you can look forward to if you decide to embrace what I have discovered.

My unexpected interactions with the metaphysical realm, and my fresh perspectives on the importance of self-created pain in our lives, are core aspects of the book and have allowed me to develop its centre-piece, which I refer to as the Arc.

This is my humble gift to my readers.

WE ARE ALL METAPHYSICAL

CHAPTER 1

Core Metaphysical Concepts

The Truth of The Universe, or God

This book gives you unashamed access to some of the forgotten truths of the way we as human beings interact with this great universe.

'God' is the aggregated light or power of the universe and is not, in my opinion, an individual entity, as some religions would have us believe. As such we are all aspects of 'God.'

There are over 300 religions in the world, and they all have their own definitions, names, and perceptions of the concept of God. In fact, according to Google, humanity has come up with around 1,000 names to describe God. Thus, while I respect the wise intent of religious institutions, and all who choose to be a part of them, it is clear that there is no mainstream consensus within religious circles on certain key spiritual aspects of life on Earth.

Don't get me wrong, I see great virtue in the power of religion to bring people together and give them a common purpose and community to enjoy. Their teachings can be very positive and loving. But, by sometimes opposing each other, rather than being more tolerant of each other, they create separation that offsets the unity they create within their own 'flocks'.

So, let us instead focus on universal awareness. Much wisdom has been lost over the centuries about the ways that we fit into the grand scheme of things in the universe. These truths cannot be found in a science laboratory or in most cases in a church, but only by accessing higher consciousness. I have been gifted with access to some of this wisdom by higher beings and I'm grateful for that.

Now it's my turn to share it with you.

This book will show you how to find a higher state of consciousness and, in turn, God's truths, for they are in fact your own truths.

What is Consciousness?

Consciousness is defined by the Cambridge Dictionary as "a state of realising and understanding something".

The Oxford Dictionary defines it as "the state of being aware and responsive to one's surroundings".

Both sources align the concept of consciousness with being aware.

However, consciousness goes deeper than that when you bring metaphysical and physical concepts into focus. Higher consciousness, including universal intelligence, is accessible through increased self-awareness. But what is the self and how can we access it?

At present, we are taught to focus largely on the mental side of ourselves, but the self that I am referring to is not found in our minds; it is felt through our bodies and interpreted *through* our minds. It is the energy and pure intelligence of our hearts or souls. It is the god-essence within us. Our hearts are our access point to our universal souls and our souls are more powerful than you can imagine.

Your full consciousness can never be thought. No matter what your ego thinks, full consciousness is ultimately impossible to experience through the mind. The conscious awareness of your soul is beyond any definition or measurement you can imagine. Using the process set out in this book, you can adopt a new practice that you can apply again and again, to bring you to higher levels of self-awareness. However, there comes a point at which the ego must fully surrender and dissolve in the knowing that your divine truth can only ever be felt and allowed to burst forth into reality. It can never be controlled by your ego.

The ancients called their female leaders goddesses, because they were believed to be beautiful, loving, intelligent, and intuitive. The truth is that we all possess these innate qualities within our true essence. Our purity cannot be thought or reasoned. It is beyond thinking. It is the energy of pure love. We all have this energy in our hearts for we *are* all it at our core.

To some, these concepts may warrant rejection because they are referenced in our vocabulary as spiritual. However, spirituality is a somewhat nebulous term and largely refers to a series of practices and mindsets that we can adopt. As I said, we are all spirits living a human existence. The only difference between a spiritual and non-spiritual person is their level of self-awareness of their own truths. The rest is semantics.

Truth and Integrity Versus Honesty

We live in a world full of honesty, but one that is often devoid of truth. We all believe in, and value, integrity, without understanding what integrity is.

Indeed, while most people would have honesty and integrity in their list of top values, we live in a world that is full of secrets and lies, many of which are described as 'little white lies.' We have collectively all fallen victim to these imposters. But why is this the case?

The concept of honesty is mind-based, and is therefore grounded in conditioning and bias. Thus, we can be expressing a view out of honesty, yet be delivering it from a preconceived mindset, which may be wrong or ill-informed. It may represent what we believe; but, as we know, beliefs can be untrue, and may not be supported by facts or realities. We may also be expressing a view from an ego state. The ego fundamentally acts to protect and project us in our lives, and is therefore often unwilling to accept or access the truth.

There are many more beliefs in this world than truths, because truth is in fact rarer than we believe. Only truth gives us the clarity of our reality and can truly dispel the confusion of our own conditioned illusions.

Integrity is derived from the concept of integration. To be *in integrity* is to be in alignment with the truth in your heart. Truth is thus found in the arms of love, not fear. Any perceived truth delivered from a place of fear is not likely to be the real truth, because it arises in the energy of conditioned thought.

In an integrated energy, your mind, soul, and body are all in synchronicity. You know what you stand for and believe in your heart, you feel it in your body, and you think and speak in alignment with these same principles. There is no separation between them.

However, since not everyone lives in alignment with the truth in their hearts, many of us have been the victims and perpetrators of deceit, particularly in relationships, including the relationship we have with ourselves.

The relationship you have with yourself is the most important relationship you will ever have, and it determines the quality and depth of all other relationships in your life.

The word 'ceit' is actually derived from a Latin word meaning to take hold of or seize. Deceit implies that we are trying to control or alter a situation, to achieve an outcome we covet. But since our motivations for achieving any outcome can also be impacted by preconceived mindsets, what we covet may also be unloving, wrong or ill-informed. Silence can also constitute a form of deceit, for in being silent we fail to express our truth when it would have been of great value to a situation. In such a place, we cannot possibly act with integrity.

The higher our level of self-awareness, however, the higher our ability to access our truths. By accessing our truths on a constant basis, we can ensure that our honest expressions are always in alignment with our inner truths.

My journey inward showed me many situations where I had lived my life in the absence of truth. I was being honest, but I was in fact being deluded by the illusions of my mind. I've been hurt and hurt others as a result. I don't hide from this reality, which was partially my own fault. I was too slow, or unable to feel into and accept the truth of many of the situations in which I found myself. I was blocked from the truth in my heart and, even if I heard it, as I know I did on occasions, I did not trust it. I lacked the self-awareness to access my truth. I tried to think my way to different outcomes that were not in alignment with my heart and therefore, love.

However, this is ultimately a no-win situation, because truth will always assert itself in the end, as I always found out. And this was often extremely painful. I was always well intended, but not well informed, because I was not really in integrity. I was not listening to the messages from my soul.

I now consider truth to be the flame that guides the way I live my life. It burns inside me with great fervour. It is the flame in which my journey to find my true self was ignited. After drowning in an ocean of disappointments, finding my truth was my quest and my saving grace.

Truth is so often the energy that ignites what is truly intended in life, so that it can come forth into reality. If you think about major events in your life, it was most likely the expression of truth by someone involved that either started, altered or ended these experiences.

The 'true-you' can be found in this same paradigm, because the true you can never be found in illusion, and the model in this book reveals the process that can help you access your truths, so they can be expressed before undue pain is inflicted on yourself or others.

In this life truth can often be punished or discarded when it comes into conflict with ego centric beliefs. However, to live without truth is energetically expensive to those who choose to do so, for the universe of which we are all a part, is infinitely aware of the intent and source of our actions, even if we are not.

Truth is inescapable and unstoppable in the end.

Truth Without the Need for Judgement

Judgement of others is the great separator in life. It even separates us from our own selves and truths. It is derived from ignorance.

Love does not judge, but it also does not hide from truth, because a life lived in the absence of truth is always based on some degree of illusion. Love and truth are the enemies of illusion and self-deception.

The need to judge others and ourselves, always stems from the absence of sufficient consciousness. It is a mask of the ego designed to lift the illusion of our own self-worth. It lives in our ego-centric minds. When we comprehend that we are all where we are meant to be, receiving the experiences in life we are meant to receive to help us grow our conscious awareness, then the need to judge others falls away, and the purity of love can take its place.

This doesn't mean that things in our lives are ideal or perfect. Perfection is, of course, rare; unless it arises in nature. When we face the truth and accept it, our ability to change for the better is possible. Just because there are problems in our lives doesn't mean we or others have failed, or are not worthy. It just means all involved have issues and concerns to attend to. They are not us – they are temporary circumstances that we can change with the right intent, if and when we face them with the integrity that is born out of respecting our truths.

Truth is the only way to enter the energy of authenticity in our lives. The higher our consciousness goes, the more we can feel compassion and gratitude for ourselves and others in any circumstances. This gives us access to greater peace and happiness and is the gateway into forgiveness and acceptance. We are all doing our best, and we are all lacking an element of self-worth in some way. This is normal, but not natural. Here lies great and latent potential for us all to grow and evolve into more loving and happy beings.

We are truly our own harshest critics. Most people are battling with their own demons and illusions, and we overstate how much they truly concern themselves with our problems. Therefore, it is important that we start our journey through truth to self-acceptance in our own hearts.

This requires the bravery to go inward first and self-reflect before we assess any circumstances. Our inner-reality will always impose itself onto our outer-reality. This is why higher self-awareness is such a critical and potent attribute to develop, and why I have taken the time to write this book. I hope my messages of love can prevent others from making the same mistakes that I have made through the absence of self-awareness in my earlier years.

Let me show you how to find this path for yourself. Your heart is begging you to be open to this journey, and to fully activate the power of love that lies inside you. This love is, and has always been, ready to be fully expressed without the limitations that fear so readily imposes upon us all. Why not participate in life from a place of higher consciousness and purity of thought?

In *Where Your Happiness Hides*, I outline how truth, love, acceptance and trust interact and iterate to allow us to break down our conditioning and move to higher levels of consciousness. All four energies are critical to embrace, if you're to find the peace that pure consciousness and presence can arise within.

Higher conscious awareness is awaiting your attention and intentions. You are worth it!

The Infinite Nature of Possibility

The universe is ever expanding and therefore everything within it must do the same. We are all an important part of this expanding universe, which is therefore not complete without any of us, and the individual light and awareness that we are.

If we can accept this – that we are an integral part of the universe – then, by definition, we must have infinite possibilities throughout the course of eternity, because the universe itself allows for infinite possibilities to arise.

This is why our conscious awareness often struggles with the possibility of failure, for it knows there is another way, because there is always another way for the universe in any situation.

This may excite you, particularly if you can perceive life as the universal soul that you are. You are truly more than your human brain could ever understand. You are pure potentiality waiting to be explored and ignited.

The Difference Between Awareness and Self-Awareness

A high sense of awareness is a powerful asset to have. It gives us intelligence and brings us opportunities in life. However, there is a fundamental difference between knowledge-based awareness and knowing-based self-awareness.

We can gain awareness by studying, reading, learning from others, and witnessing the world around us. Schools teach us the mental awareness of concepts that the world thinks we should know or that we choose to learn. At university, we choose the types of concepts we want to understand, so that we can build a successful career. Awareness can sometimes be seen as an achievement, since it involves effort to learn, and gives you IQ or Intelligence Quotient. IQ is largely a measure of your ability to reason and is derived from your mind.

However, awareness is different to self-awareness. Self-awareness allows you to become the true you because by definition it entails you knowing yourself. It gives you II, or Intuitive Intelligence, which is not taught in most of society's learning structures, including most families in western societies.

Psychologists refer to Emotional Intelligence or EQ, but this is somewhat different to II. EQ refers to your ability to sense into and interpret the emotions of others or yourself. However, this sensing and interpretation may still be done through distorted belief structures with which the receiver is not in touch. These may distort the conclusions that are reached.

The world is at the early stages of embarking on a journey into Artificial Intelligence or AI. My concern is that this new tool may take us further away from a world where II is a common trait of human beings.

The quest for greater awareness *can* help you find self-awareness, for it can instigate and assist your journey. Gaining awareness is often a doing process, whereas the journey to self-awareness is primarily an allowing process.

In this process, your ego gets out of the way of your consciousness establishing itself within you, and it becomes a journey managed by love in the energy of surrender. It is done best by not trying to achieve an end outcome, but by letting your soul determine your path and how far you go, for it knows you infinitely and intimately. Your heart is the seat of your intuition and knows the truth of you better than your mind ever will.

When you move towards your intuition, you are effectively moving into higher universal consciousness. This is an energetic experience and cannot originate in your head, as it surpasses mind-based understandings.

I made the mistake in the earlier years of my awakening of being too controlling, determined to achieve enlightenment at all costs, and I found it hard to surrender to my evolving self-awareness and effectively 'get out of the way' to enable my own expansion to take place. Looking back, I now know that I slowed down my progress with such a controlling attitude.

Now that I have substantially mastered the energy of allowing, I know that following the Arc can assist those on a self-awareness path, and this is particularly so once they have learned to keep their minds out of the 'cockpit', and switch on the autopilot that lies within them.

This act of surrendering is often difficult because our minds love to be in control. This is normal, for they are wrongly conditioned to believe that they are the primary source of our consciousness.

In the process of increasing your self-awareness, feelings can be a gateway through which you can know your real truth, for real truth naturally comes from our hearts and is sensed through our bodies. It cannot be thought until after it is felt, then interpreted by our minds.

Our thoughts can be influenced by the conditioning in our minds. This can influence the way we feel. Interpreting our feelings on a constant basis is, therefore, a key aspect of our journey to our truth.

Unfortunately, most parents do not encourage their children to know the truth of themselves. How could they when they don't even know the truth of *themselves*?

This wisdom of how to discover the true-you, has been dismissed through centuries of human conditioning. As a rule, we are taught and shown who to be, not how to find the truth of *what* and who we are. We believe we must meet the expectations of the world around us, not create our own world and be the centre of our own universe, even if this defies our true essence as creators.

I do not stand in judgement of others by making these statements. For most of my life, I lived the same way and even raised my children, in their younger years, in alignment with such societal norms.

But finding our way to this truth has become a lost art and it is causing us great collective pain and suffering, which we do not need to experience. It has left us in a state of mass-confusion and ignorance, because much of what we think about ourselves is in fact illusory. To some extent we are told what to be and how to think in this world, but unfortunately the journey inward to our own realities is not well sign posted. It has become a kind of mystery.

In ancient civilisations, such as Egypt, there were what were called Mystery Schools, set up to teach the elite and leadership classes how to undertake this journey to higher conscious awareness. Our so-called modern world has largely lost sight of these principles and the associated wisdom is largely found in non-mainstream literature and organisations of a 'spiritual' nature.

As human beings, we want to fit in of course, be loved and be successful. As a result, we typically follow the leaders around us, including our parents, so that we can feel safe, accepted and secure. We are conditioned to look outward for validation and love in our lives, not to go inward where our real truths and self-worth can only ever be felt and sourced. Our greatest fear is to fail and, therefore, reinforce our deep-seated fear that we are not lovable. However, ultimately we are trying to avoid a fear that has absolutely no validity, for we are loved by the universe, and our own souls.

The power of higher self-awareness is immense, because knowing your true self allows you to face the world with authenticity and integrity. From here you can live the life that your heart yearns for you to live. In this energy, you are clear about what is of interest and value to you as a person. Confusion is replaced by clarity in this wonderful place. Your fears melt away in the cauldron of your own self-love.

Without this connection to your truth, you are likely to feel the constant pain of trying to navigate your way through life, doing things you might like or even tolerate, but not love. Thinking your way through life is often a zero-sum game.

I have lived both paths. Eventually, I remembered how to go about discovering the true me. For the first 57 years of my life, I pursued the things I thought I was meant to pursue, until I worked out what I really liked. I excelled at and put my time and energy into activities I moderately liked but didn't really love. And I did many things to satisfy those around me, particularly the people I trusted and thought had more wisdom than me, like my parents.

I didn't trust my own judgement or desires, but how could I – I couldn't even connect to them, because I was oblivious to where I could find them.

The 'pipe' I naturally had – and could use to connect to the truth of myself – had become closed and cluttered by my preconditioned beliefs about how I should live my life.

But who was going to clear that pipe, so I could connect to the truth of me, and discover what I was capable of being?

There was only one answer to that question: it was me. No one else could do that for me. Only I had exclusive access to my heart and my feelings that would ultimately guide me home.

I did have guidance from learned beings and mentors to show me the way to find my truth, without whom my advancement would have been slower; but they could only shine their lights to guide me forward along the path. I had to walk that path myself, sometimes in the light and sometimes in the dark. I held the hands of those willing to help, but my feet were the ones taking the steps, experiencing the highs and lows of the journey, and taking me step-by-step towards acknowledging and embracing my true self. Sometimes I stumbled and fell on the uneven (and what often seemed to be unfair) cobblestones of life, but I never gave up.

The journey home to YOU is the greatest journey you can take, if you choose it. Your truth, once you discover it, will show you much, and release you from pain and mediocrity as you move towards greater self-love and peace in your life and away from the illusions that currently control your thinking, and are always temporary in nature, because the universe will always dissolve illusions in the end.

There is no risk in this journey because ultimately you are striving to become something you already are. There may be emotional releases as you follow your path, but all this is, is illusion being dissolved. The love you seek is inside you already, and the truth of yourself is waiting to come forth, once you remove the veil of conditioning that is stopping your true self from bursting forth into your human reality.

What awaits you on the other side is a life with minimal pain, which is far more fleeting than you currently know, and sources of happiness and fulfilment which you most likely cannot yet perceive.

The 'University of Life'

The universe is an ever-expanding energetic field constituted by light, and we are all just a fractal of light within this enormous field. The field has no limits. Accordingly, therefore, neither do we. Our journeys will never end, and our learnings will never cease.

As a fractal of light, we are individual and unique yet connected to all the other fractals. This is a bit like a string of lights. Only the brightness or frequency of each fractal varies in intensity.

Although we are a part of this fascinating continuum – a continuum beyond the comprehension of the human mind – scientists strive to understand how the universe works and how it arose, and we must salute them for trying. However, this is an intellectual impossibility beyond the workings of our three-dimensional intelligence or IQ, unless we can access the infinite intelligence that enlightenment brings.

We live in the third dimension physically, but our souls can access so much more if we allow them to, by 'clearing the pipe' I referred to above. This is a big part of the enlightenment process that can bring forth your halo and the light in the centre of your chest, just like the pictures of Jesus Christ and his mother Mary in many Christian churches.

Our souls are all at different stages of journeying to enlightenment, vibrating at different pitches and in different dimensions. Any reference you may have heard about 'racing' to the gates of heaven is incorrect, for it is not a race but a never-ending journey of wonderful discovery that we all share together.

As wiser souls than me have espoused, you can never storm the gates of heaven and force your way in – you must earn the keys to the locks. This reflects the different journeys of expansion we are all here to experience at the behest of divine timing. Increased enlightenment and wisdom are primarily the by-products of experience, not thinking.

Therefore, to progress we must truly understand, then overcome our issues in reality. Evolution is a gradual process that cannot be rushed.

Life is truly living us, we are not living it, and as we experience different lifetimes and different incarnations, our souls ascend through the different dimensions in a way commensurate with the vast experiences they orchestrate.

The current life you are living is just one of the many incarnations within which your soul is expressing itself, for the purpose of expansion and evolution. They are all unfolding concurrently, and they can all change the energy within each other.

Ironically, our souls never left what we call heaven, we just think they have. And this is a great truth we need to remember. We were never separated from God, from the universe. Our eternal connection is ever present within us, even though we are temporarily in a physical form. The day you become perfect in the eyes of 'God' is the day your current incarnation on this Earth will end. You will die. So, there is no rush! The ultimate consequences of attaining perfection are quite severe from a purely physical perspective!

The 'university of life' teaches us, through the course of our lives, who we truly are; yet a great part of this journey is first to discover what and who we are not: to dispel the illusory and conditioned thoughts we have been taught to believe are true.

To know this, we must first let go of our misguided beliefs. Then the universe will show you what you are capable of being: *not* just a human *doing* activities, but rather a human *being* pure love, and discovering all that that can bring forth for you and the world you inhabit.

CHAPTER 2

Controls Over Our Fate

A Place of Choice and Decision

Many people believe in fate, or in other words that a higher power controls what happens in our lives. Others might call this destiny. Many of these people inherently believe there is a universal force, or God directing our core outcomes.

At the other extreme, many people believe that life is random, and therefore humans have total freedom to choose what they want, that there are no divine forces at play, and there is unlikely to be any life after death.

The real answer is that we co-create with divine forces. It's a complex hybrid of the two opposite perspectives stated above, resulting in the Earth being a place of choice and decision, with consequences for all we decide to bring into reality. What ultimately matters in terms of determining the outcomes in our lives, is the source of intelligence from which we choose: our egoic minds or our loving hearts.

We are all connected to the universal field through our hearts. This connects us to an infinite source of intelligence that is ever-present throughout our eternal journey. Consider our hearts to be like a portal to the internet. Our hearts are the portal to our powerful souls. The ancient Egyptians, who had much spiritual wisdom, used to refer to them as the under-soul and over-soul respectively, such was their connection.

Our soul knows more about us than we know about ourselves and is therefore worthy of our trust.

It knows:

- our divine plan for this life,
- what we came here to learn and overcome,
- who we will love,
- what we need,
- what we believe,
- what we fear,
- what our attachments are,
- what our karma is, and
- what lives we have previously lived and will live in the future.

In fact, the universal field knows more than that. It knows everything about everything in this universe, and all this wisdom is recorded in what is called the Akashic Records. Within these records, there is complete knowing about everything. There are no limits.

Each time you die, the light within you – which is your light being, higher self or life force – returns to the universal field, remembers what your metaphysical amnesia has hidden from you, and has full access to divine energies and records. In the metaphysical, there is access to all knowledge and you are omni-present. There, you can survive for eternity without a mind or body.

However, there are some among us who can consciously access the Akashic Records, in their present 3D lives on Earth, and they can see what we call the past, present and future. Seers, like Nostradamus, have been known to do this, for they have a dimensional capacity to see into this universal database.

Others can access it subconsciously. Indeed, whenever you choose from your intuition or heart, you are making choices in alignment with this infinite or higher sources of intelligence.

This is possible for all of us to do regularly once we reach a high enough level of evolution or vibration. It just takes practice, intention and the will of God.

But what do I mean by vibration and why does it matter?

Our vibration in this life is defined by the rate at which our body cells and energy fields oscillate and vibrate. Everything on Earth and beyond has a vibration, even a rock, for all is light or energy. The more in tune with positive energies and higher consciousness we become, the lighter we feel, as our vibration rises.

The Arc, which is set out in later chapters of this book, defines a tried and tested way of expanding our conscious awareness and bringing you closer to aligning with higher energetic frequencies in this life. By gradually raising your vibration, you can essentially move away from living in a state of fear and move more into the energy of love. The vibration of love is the foundation for accessing and working with higher forms of intelligence, including you own, beyond the third dimension. But, more than that, it gives you the possibility of greater happiness and joy, for the lighter you are the happier you will be. It's that simple.

It's About Time

Let's consider time in this context of our unfolding or awakening. The reality is: there is no such thing as time at a universal level, because time is a man-made concept, used by humans to make life on Earth more practical. It was introduced to Earth by Thoth, a wise being who walked the Earth in ancient times. In this way, time is merely the passing of human thought, referenced to the Earth's relativity to the Sun.

But the universe doesn't work off time, it works off the coalescing of universal energies such as light and love, which move at their own speed. The universe knows of our human obsession with time, but ignores it, for time (as we define it) is not relevant anywhere else in the universe.

In many circumstances, therefore, focussing on time in your awakening can be counterproductive. There is no point setting the universe deadlines, because deadlines go outside the energetic flows of nature. Putting a deadline on the universe is an act of ignorance. It is better to be in sync with the energy of every individual moment and react accordingly.

Our minds, of course, constantly seek to move faster than nature itself. This can cause us great pain, as we want events to occur at a different pace to what is energetically possible, or what is likely or destined to unfold.

Probability is key in this, because there are multiple dimensions, and we all have multiple universes we can experience, in which events can occur at all kinds of speeds, depending on the choices we make.

The universe is so complex and is, in truth, beyond the comprehensive powers of the human brain!

But what I have been told by my metaphysical mentors is that, once something has happened in the physical, it is done and recorded in the Akashic Records, and our present and so-called futures are all recorded in the records based on probabilities. Just as the energies associated with events in the past can change, according to our perspective of them, these probabilities of the future can also change. The universe is a dynamic field of energy that is constantly in flow and transforming itself.

The setting of time frames is therefore insignificant and fraught with the painful experience of disappointment. Most of us cannot tell the future – unless we are sufficiently evolved to access the Akashic Records to see what is probable in that future – but even if we could, we would only witness probabilities, not certainties.

Consider this: Albert Einstein is regarded as one of the most intelligent people that ever lived. His IQ was estimated at 215. The universe is infinite. Hardly a competition, don't you think?

How Do I Align with My Destiny?

What does this all mean for your life and your so-called destiny?

If you constantly choose and manifest outcomes from your egoic mind, you will make choices outside of the flow of the natural universal forces to which you are subject, and of which you are ultimately a part. When we choose through our egos, we are prone to make decisions with a separation mindset, causing the possibility of great pain in our lives as we diverge from our intended paths. We will usually seek security and safety over fun and adventure.

Only your heart and the universal field knows whether your choices are in proper alignment with your divine intentions. If they are not, the universe may create synchronicity to effectively dismantle them, bringing you the learnings that you need to experience to bring you home to the love in your heart. It does this through you, for you, not to you.

This interference is why people use expressions like, "it will be, what it will be" and "it will unfold". This wisdom is correctly aligned with the reality that we are all subject to the universal forces that reside within us and are all around us. These powers are immense should they act to alter your unfolding life.

Such actions are for a good purpose – to realign you with the universe itself and give you every opportunity to grow and expand.

The universe does have a hierarchy, in some ways like our so-called modern organisations. It operates with intent and, essentially, we are not alone in our endeavours in each life we live.

There are currently 12 dimensions that we work our way up through. As we evolve and our vibrations rise, we take on higher dimensional experiences and responsibilities.

There are also higher beings who are the custodians of different aspects of universal existence and gatherings of beings that make decisions in the interests of civilisations. These higher beings are pure light and love, like we become when we die; though they can manifest into the physical should they choose to, like Jesus and Buddha did, and may have done so in other forms not as familiar to us.

Higher beings are omnipresent and active in universal activities. This means that they can be present in multiple places and dimensions at once. Archangel Metatron is the custodian of the Akashic Records. There is a body of twelfth dimensional beings called the Council of Light that directs aspects of the universe. There is a high vibrational council called the Galactic Council that oversees the Earth and other civilisations across our galaxy. Yes, Star Wars is more accurate than you think! And we all have spirit guides that oversee our lives and interact with our souls to assist with our unfoldings. We are not alone!

How do I know this? I have interacted with them all, as have others.

I can see into other dimensions and have accessed the Akashic Records to witness some of my concurrent lives in meditation, however there are people around who at present have far greater energies than me in this regard.

I know that these kinds of psychic abilities are the capability of source in form, which we all are. You most likely have this capability, should you believe in it and choose to explore it!

These energies want you to grow and expand forever, as does your soul. The universe will therefore give you what you need in life, until you make choices that align with your heart's desires or wants. However, giving you what you need may not always be pleasant. And by 'need' we refer to your need to expand and learn.

This is how awakenings occur. If your soul chooses for your awareness and self-awareness to expand, events in your life are likely to support new perspectives by encouraging you to alter your belief structures and live more from love. Painful events are normally the catalyst for such awakenings, like a death or relationship failure.

Many people are awakening at this time in our evolutionary cycle, for the energies on the Earth are of a higher vibration and are now more aligned with showing humanity its truths and supporting us to transition to higher dimensions. Love is effectively imposing itself on our lives with more power and rising vibrations and will be the dominant energy of the future on Earth. Resistance to this can, and most likely will, cause you pain.

You can either learn from this pain and expand through it or continue to experience suffering arising from a low vibration or fearful existence.

So, we can make choices, but the universe, through your soul, has both the power and intelligence to override these choices if they are not in alignment with the love and truth in your own heart. Your timing may also not be in alignment with the intentions of universal energies. Accordingly, your expected timings, as to when some things may occur, such as meeting the love of your life or getting that dream job, can prove to be inaccurate. That lover or dream job may not be ready for you when you demand it. Gently asking for the things you want with no demands for when they arrive is the key to co-creating with infinite intelligence.

This is why the power of intentions, that I discuss in another chapter, is so important. Loving intentions bring you in sync with love. This the universe will support whole-heartedly by creating opportunities for you to step into.

Your heart knows what is in your best interests and why you chose to come to Earth in this life. Your ego is clueless in this regard, unless it has downloaded this information from your heart.

As humans we tend to think that matter is all that really matters, and that time should rule our lives. These beliefs block our true understanding of the truth of our existence and hold us in the vice of mind-based hopes and expectations. They block our ability to access our full capabilities, and to discover our true possibilities. They also keep us out of alignment with nature. Most things will never unfold until they are energetically ready to do so.

It is important to recognise that all is energy. Accordingly, we are surrounded by possibilities in our periphery and these all have their own energies, which can ignite when we are energetically in alignment with them.

That's why I say that expectations can be the enemy of fun and possibility. After all, love is the creator of infinite possibilities, and you are love at your core, making you a natural creator. You have love inside you, and you are love intrinsically. Relying solely on your mind and its propensity to set expectations and plans to direct your life, takes you out of sync with universal potentialities and the natural rhythms of life.

The Arc, as I explain in later chapters, gives you a natural way to access higher consciousness and to give yourself the opportunity to live in alignment with infinite intelligence. Everything we do impacts on our physical and metaphysical realities concurrently. That is what we inherently are. To think otherwise is to live from ignorance, not true intelligence.

The Arc is a natural way that allows you to make choices that are in flow with love, and your divine interests. Who would not want that?

The simple answer is that many people do not understand what is possible, because they have never been taught these kinds of realities. Ignorance has been described as bliss by humanity, but the truth is that it is holding us back from experiencing the real bliss we were born to experience. This is a shame, but we have nothing else to blame but our limited awareness of WHAT we all truly are.

Exploring the Arc, *remembering* it and applying it, or your version of it, can take you to real bliss in this life. It's yours if you want it. Come with me on this journey if you choose to bravely step forward!

CHAPTER 3

The Vibrational Power of Nature

We Are Nature

We are truly immersed in love. It is our core energy, and it is all around us, although I know this is hard to believe at times, given the negative events that we often witness in this world. It does however, bear witness to what is possible, when humanity finds its own truth en masse.

The truth is that all hearts are connected by love. There are no exceptions to this. Unfortunately, our minds have other ideas and so we judge each other continuously, believing that we are totally separate beings.

When I meditate and activate my third eye, I often go into oneness and witness it for real. Everything that is natural turns pure white when I open my eyes, and is connected to each other like a big white spider web, or like being in a cloud in a plane.

Such experiences have shown me the reality that is espoused in spiritual literature: that we are all one. This truth is out of step with mainstream thinking.

Nature is a pure energy that we can merge with to advance our self-awareness journey. Nature is high vibration for it is light, and it can assist you to get in touch with your truth. In a place of nature, there is less interference or distractions from the outside world, which assists you to be able to hear the messages intended for you from your soul.

We are nature and not separate from it, so the truth is that your connection to nature already exists. You always have the opportunity to open and allow nature to more consciously and intentionally merge with your energies.

The elements of the Earth are vibrating at the vibration of unconditional love, for they are a component of Mother Nature and connected to her consciousness. We may think of this planet as a rock floating in space and being in orbit with other physical bodies, including the Sun, but it is much more than that. It is alive in pure consciousness. The same goes for the other galactic bodies in the universe we are a part of, including the Sun that warms us.

Think of the sunlight that warms us, the air we breathe, the water in our great oceans and rivers, and the soil and forests all around us. They are all vibrationally high – unless humanity has polluted and distorted their purity – and they are all around us. We are a part of nature and not separate from it at all. We truly are the same light or vibration. It's just that this energy of love must be stepped down because our bodies cannot hold the full power that other entities can, like the Earth, or the Sun.

There are three core ways you can work with these natural energies to help you undertake the natural evolutionary processes of the Arc.

1. Be In Nature

Firstly, when you are trying to hear the messages of your soul in a process I call conscious receptivity, you will be able to tune in far better in a natural environment that you love. For me that is on a beach, on my farm, or high on a mountain in the bush. The beach is one of the highest vibrational places on the Earth, because in this place the five key elements of the Earth intersect – namely earth (i.e. rocks and sand), fire (i.e. the sunlight), air, water, and spirit (i.e. other universal energies). Mountains are also extremely high vibration, given the clean air and water that is often found there, and are often extremely uplifting because of the views they allow you to be inspired by. Of course, you will have your own beautiful place in nature where you feed relaxed, at home and at peace. All of nature is of a high vibration.

The Earth and the Sun are great vibrational forces in our lives. The Sun is more than a large gaseous object that emits heat and electromagnetic rays. Sunlight is pure love and much of our consciousness is brought into our hearts through this energy. After conception, our consciousness enters us through the Sun. Our minds don't witness the energy of the Sun, but our souls are in deep connection with the rest of the universe and this light.

Did you know that communicating with the Sun allows you to use its loving light rays to heal you. *I use it a lot, for it is the same energy as my soul, only in a stepped-up version.* Of course, too much sunlight can harm our bodies, so our exposure needs to be managed sensibly.

I discuss the healing energies of nature in another part of this book.

Moonlight is another, less intense version of sunlight as it represents sunlight reflecting onto the Earth from the moon. This is why many spiritual people meditate and conduct rituals in times of full moons. But you will never get sunburnt in the moonlight, which makes it easier to spend time in protracted meditation and self-reflection.

Many spiritual people use crystals to increase the vibrational energy around them as well as allow them to tune in to the universe, including their own souls. We often use or hear the expression 'crystal clear' in our vocabulary. These beautiful and natural stones, emit frequencies that contain wisdom for our souls. They possess pure consciousness. Radios use crystal technologies to receive and transmit the frequencies that form into radio shows. These realities I appreciate can be hard to believe, but it is another truth we have largely forgotten.

2. Nature Is Intelligent

Secondly, nature is a great teacher when we simply learn from its many beautiful attributes. When we observe how it operates, we see instinct and consciousness in full swing. Only humanity can distort these natural flows out of ignorance, because of the commonly held belief that we are above nature and not a part of it. Nature is comprised of pure intelligence, constantly evolving and rebalancing. What is more ignorant us or nature? Take some time to feel into that question with your heart. The answer may surprise you.

My book *Show Me the Harmony*, contains an entire chapter on this topic!

3. Nature Is Cleansing

Thirdly, places in nature of high vibration provide a means by which our energy fields can be cleansed of negative energies that are ready to be released back into the universe.

I regularly swim in the ocean and set my intention that the energies in the sunlight, sand, air, and waters cleanse and clear any negative energies in my field that can be released at that time.

Certain places on the Earth which have been the location for high vibrational ceremonies and events are often referred to in spiritual circles as sacred sites. Attending these locations with a positive intent to release past pain can assist you to remove negative beliefs and vibrations that are ready to be set free from your being. This happens naturally when you are in attendance with the right intentions.

In 2019, I personally attended a series of sacred sites in Egypt, the United Kingdom, Hawaii, New Zealand, and Australia to process karma at sites of significance to my universal thread. My experiences in each location were profound, bringing forth new levels of self-awareness and the processing of energies I was ready to release.

An important part of the Arc is deep self-reflection. This means going inward without the interference of the ego, but with the assistance of a mind willing to assist in the process objectively. Self-reflection is an art we can all master, and that is so important if you want to enhance your self-awareness. Being in nature amps up the clarity of feedback that can emerge in a self-reflection process, such as meditation.

Next time you are in nature, breathe in the air, feel the soil under your feet, feel the warmth of the sun on your skin and marvel at any water and trees that are gracing your presence. In this beautiful place, feel into your inner beauty and enquire about questions and feelings that arise through your consciousness and body. The answers will be forthcoming and pure, just like the elements you are experiencing.

Listen and trust what you hear!

CHAPTER 4

Our Vibrational Connectivity

We Are All One

As I touched on earlier, it is normal for most of humanity to believe in separation, and maintain a separation consciousness, because our egos teach us that we are separate from each other and only connected if we choose to be. Entrenched in this is the belief that life is competitive, that we have all been sent to this rock to die, and who knows what happens after that.

But none of this is true. Not only is separation an impossibility in metaphysical realms, but we are all eternal. We live on after death, connected forever.

I can attest to that because I can witness beings beyond this physical plane and do so every day.

The universe is a big ball or stream of light. We are all therefore light beings. We are all separate fractals of one big continuum of light – we just have different vibrational levels, which reflect our different stages of evolution. We are all connected through this light to each other, and every other fractal of light in the universe, which means everything, because everything is light.

Our level of evolution is just a timing difference. We are all on the same eternal journey. Different souls have been created at different 'times', for want of a better word, and have had different experiences or learning opportunities.

As I mentioned earlier, the metaphysical realm currently comprises of 12 dimensions; but this number will expand for eternity. As we grow, we progress to higher dimensions; thus, the person we are represented as, in this current life, is not necessarily a reflection of our true dimensional vibration levels. This is because we reincarnate to face different challenges and have different experiences. Thus, in some lives, you may be a leader, a pauper, a soldier, or a billionaire. We all receive the experiences we need to expand up through the dimensions. This process never ends. Once we have learned our lessons and escaped the karmic cycle, we can choose if we return to this planet or not. This is referred to as becoming an Ascended Master.

The place we often refer to as heaven is actually a metaphysical hierarchy of different dimensions of light. It is not a physical place, as we may have been led to believe. After death, our souls return and remain there, for they are omnipresent, meaning they can go anywhere in the universe faster than the speed of light. Truly it is beyond the comprehension of our minds.

I once had an experience of having my consciousness teleported to the star cluster called the Pleaides. You can see it in the night sky. This is 444 light years from Earth. My journey to this planet took what felt like a few seconds.

Such connections are possible, because we are all universal beings of the same source, returning to the same place after death on Earth, not separate beings. Understanding this is core to grasping why our world is so full of human interactions that are not positive.

The day we understand *en masse* that we are on the same team, energetically connected and needing each other to evolve and survive, is the day that this world can start to improve from its current situation. And this will be assisted when we all take responsibility for our individual pains and learn to go inward rather than blame the people around us for our problems. Those around us are helping us to receive the lessons we came here to receive, even that jilted lover you now despise!

We are universal for we are part of the universe. Unity consciousness is our future, once we concede to reality.

Karma is well documented on the Earth, and has been in place for centuries. It relates to us being all one and interconnected, such that when we do something to another fractal of light, we effectively do it to ourselves; and feel it too. Such actions impact all in the universal field. Karma will come, as is often said, because ultimately it must, until we collectively enter a higher dimensional state as our universal selves. At this point, it can be released quickly by us.

We can all *reintroduce* karma if we act inappropriately. However, at higher vibrations this need not wait until our future lives to be rebalanced, if we know how to undertake the process of release.

To be released from the karmic cycle is just a choice, which is now available to us all. The era of karma is coming to an end in the higher energies or vibrations that we are currently alive within (and in fact already are). But to release ourselves from karma, as it stands, requires our commitment to higher consciousness. This is a choice like everything in our lives. This occurs as we go to higher vibrational dimensions while we are alive. Here, we can live only from the vibrational wisdom and energy of love, all balanced within the big ball of light that we call the universe.

Those who do not choose to extract themselves from the karmic cycle will remain trapped within it and continue to experience its forces, both in this life and in future lives upon the Earth plane.

In Egypt, after visiting a temple, I experienced bleeding from several parts of my body, including my genitals. My bed the next morning looked like a crime scene! I later found out from my mentors that I restated karma created by one of my incarnations in Ancient Egypt in the 25th century BC, relating to sexual impropriety. This showed me that time may tick by, but energy remains present in other dimensions.

So, how we treat each other goes way beyond just our own lives. As one beam of light, represented by different fractals, what we do, and even energetically think or project at others, impacts upon the whole of humanity and beyond.

Together we are one beam of light. Our role in that beam is to *be* the truth of what we are. We were all created as part of the whole. You can never separate yourself from this truth, and you are dearly loved within it.

The Spirit Realm

Our fear of the metaphysical realms is widespread, with most believing it does not exist or in a state of uncertainty. Some people are curious about and seek to connect with it, though those who express their interest publicly are often condemned for believing in it, and in some centuries have been persecuted or put to death – persecuted by ignorance. This rises from the prevalence of conditioned beliefs on this subject. We do not generally wish to believe in something that we cannot prove – even though we are metaphysical and physical simultaneously. In a sense, we fear what we really are out of ignorance.

I respect all opinions on this subject, but I have my own opinion that I will never change. The universe has proven to me beyond any doubt that life exists beyond the grave and that we reincarnate eternally. I'm sure many readers have had their own experiences or are curious to understand it more closely. The fact that you are reading this book probably means you have an open mind to these truths and are ready to explore them further.

The metaphysical has presented itself to me in the following ways over the last 10 years:

- *I have had apparitions or visitations of many non-physical beings, including elementals, Archangels Michael and*

Metatron, Jesus, Hathor and Thoth, just to name a few. Beings from Sirius and the Pleaides are regular visitors in my home. These visitations are commonplace in my life – so much so that I'm not sure who or what many of them are. I just enjoy their presence.
- *I see and feel non-physical beings, including those commonly known as ghosts. I have learned to remove those I don't want to interact with.*
- *My dead parents and grandparents visit me periodically.*
- *I have had well over 150 significant out-of-body experiences and metaphysical happenings that I have recorded. There are too many to discuss in this book.*
- *I have talked to other universal beings directly, but also through the assistance of a channeler of universal wisdom and psychic professionals that I trust.*
- *I have had the gift of miracle healings of my body through the love of metaphysical beings, principally from the Pleaides.*
- *By progressively applying the Arc over the last nine years, I am now in direct connection with my own consciousness or soul. It teaches me new insights every day and opens me to new metaphysical experiences that I am ready to have.*

I use the word 'psychic' in this book as it is a commonly used phrase to describe someone or something that is linked in some way to metaphysical forces or energies. The Oxford dictionary refers to psychic phenomena as being "not possible according to natural laws". I'm sure that readers, like me, who have had their own metaphysical experiences, will know how natural such phenomena are, even if it is virtually impossible to prove to others that they have taken place.

I was always curious about the metaphysical growing up. I loved a great walk through a cemetery or watching a ghost movie. My experiences with the metaphysical have been almost exclusively positive and loving. I have had about ten active ghosts in my home.

However, as a reiki master, I became trained to manage these metaphysical realms. They do not scare me – they excite me. I'm one of them, after all, I just have a body.

Hollywood movies are wide off the mark and scare us unnecessarily about the spirit realm. The spirit realm respects the principal of free will. If you tell a ghost to stay away from your field and not harm you it will from my experiences.

I once had a ghost attach itself to me and come with me from Hiroshima in Japan to Australia. The spirit told me that he died in the 1945 nuclear blast. He showed me what it was like to be suspended and trapped in no man's land between heaven and Earth. It was a terrible place with little light and low energy. That feeling haunted me for months.

I returned him to the place from whence he came. I was told he was not ready to be passed over to heaven as yet. I shall leave that to greater powers than I.

The point is that, like it or not, we live in a soup of energy. It is all around us. I am just fortunate that I see, hear, and feel metaphysical energies as I do. I believe that my lack of fear of it brings it into my periphery. I enjoy it and all it teaches me.

The metaphysical realm is full of love and is not, as we have come to believe, out to get us. It is generally supportive and loving and there are many ways to access its loving guidance.

Given we are all at different points of evolution, there are of course many people who are more advanced than me in these metaphysical fields.

But, by applying a process like the Arc, you too can connect more with the metaphysical. Our souls are metaphysical, they are our eternal selves, and through it we can all potentially access the wisdom of the universe.

When we sleep at night, our consciousness invariably visits other dimensions, particularly the fourth dimension. We are very much connected to such dimensional realms and can interact with them when our minds do not shut down our truths out of fear.

Thus, we can all interact with the metaphysical more consciously if we choose to. It's the birthright of all human beings in form. I have, and many of the beliefs and views that I put forward in this book, that are not mainstream thinking, have come from my many interactions with beings beyond this world. It has been a great gift to my awareness and self-awareness.

I know many readers may not accept this information, and I am compassionate to that sensitivity.

Our Galactic Connections

Humanity has a belief that it is alone in the universe. This belief is not true. We harbour a fear of life beyond Earth. because it is all we let ourselves know. This is an illusion we need to dispel, because meaningful connection with beings from other dimensions and locations beyond the Earth is possible. Who knows what they could teach us if we let them!

Many Hollywood movies have demonised what we call Unidentified Flying Objects (UFOs), and through countless movies, they have reinforced the human belief that aliens will one day come to Earth and try to destroy our civilisation. But we have no basis to believe this notion. In fact, there is more evidence to the contrary. There are many recorded sightings of UFOs, many ancient temples and stories mention interactions with beings from beyond the Earth, yet how many times have they attacked our cities?

I know that we are not alone, because I have had a number of visitations from, and discussions with, beings from other parts of our galaxy. There has been nothing, but love expressed in these experiences and concern for the welfare of humanity and me. I too was fearful at first of these events, because of my human conditioning, but I have let this go now.

It is interesting that, in recent years, governments around the world are being more honest about interactions with so-called UFOs. Even the US Congress has discussed it openly with the military and CIA. Finally, we are allowing greater levels of truth on these matters.

One day, I believe our brothers and sisters from these other places will make themselves more known to us as a broader population. I eagerly look forward to that day!

The Earth and its inhabitants are connected to the broader universe and all beings that exist within it. We are all one and, accordingly, the vibrations generated on this planet influence the vibrational resonance of the galaxy and universe we exist within.

Many of us have lived lives in other parts of the universe, and as a result we have subconscious memories and connections to these places.

I have a deep connection to Sirius, and have been told by my metaphysical mentors that this is my star-seed connection. You can witness Sirius as a bright star in the night sky.

Almost certainly you too will have a deep connection to other parts of this great universe.

Our world does have many unfortunate and low vibrational aspects to it. Many human interactions are less than ideal and are derived from our ego centric way of being. In many cultures its every man and woman for themselves.

Of course, there are beautiful souls and wonderful places where harmony exists between people.

I recently visited a nation I would put into this category in Western Samoa. I have never experienced such a harmonious and united nation as this country, and I applaud them for how they live their lives as a collective.

Although the Earth is an experiment and a place of choice and decision, where we can live from love or fear, and make choices every day on which vibration we align with; many other places in the universe are of a higher vibration, where love is the collectively chosen way. As the Earth is third dimensional, it is of a relatively low vibration and levels of intelligence, compared to many other parts of the universe.

However, being a civilisation of density does allow us to have some wonderful experiences you may not be able to experience in worlds where all is light. Sex is the best example that comes to mind.

One day, my hope is that humanity will come to understand its vibrational connection to the rest of our galaxy and the entire universe that we exist within, including other dimensions. Until then, humanity as a collective will continue to have deep fears of many manifestations that we can't explain, largely because we are not truly curious about them – we are in fear.

I have been fortunate enough to debunk many of these core fears of humanity through my own experiences for my own sake. Many of these experiences were not solicited by my mind and just occurred through synchronicity. They came to me. I did not seek them.

Knowing that there is a universe out there, which I intrinsically belong to, has helped me to embrace my universal self and relax more into life. For starters, my fear of death is no more, for I know it is just a passageway to the ultimate in new beginnings for me as a being. Death, like birth, is something that most of us have mastered many times over in our universal threads, probably hundreds of times. It's on our natural path.

I have also explored many of my past lives in my quest to find my true self. I am grateful to the enlightened people who have helped me to do this. These experiences have enabled me to piece together much of the karma that has been foundational to my core fears in this life, and I have thankfully applied the Arc to remove or temper them.

Heaven and Hell

We constantly refer to notions of heaven and hell, and wonder if they exist. Hell does not, although I understand that there are low vibrational parts of the universe that are best avoided by our souls, some of which are on Earth. But why do we think we need to die to experience heaven?

Heaven is available right here, right now, to those who open to the truth of their being and the word of God, and are ready to enjoy the journey to higher consciousness. All it takes is opening to the vibration of love that you already are!

Heaven on Earth is yours to be experienced in its fullness right now, if you want it. Most don't want it because they have never been told that it is possible. That's not their fault, they were led to believe until now that it wasn't something they could experience until they die.

What needs to die is our egos, so that we can allow our full connection to love to take over the life that we are in. In this place our light beings can come into a better balance with, and two-way awareness of, our human beings. This is where true peace can be found, and heaven on Earth becomes our reality.

Trusting in Your Inner-Wisdom

When most people start on their self-awareness journey, and delve into spiritual concepts, they have a natural tendency to look beyond the power of their own heart for divine guidance. I have observed this in even advanced spiritual people.

I did it too, for several years.

The presence and existence of high vibrational beings has been well documented by religions and other sources over the centuries. These high vibrational beings watch over us and love us dearly as I outlined above.

Through metaphysical channelling experiences I have talked with many of them many times.

Their love for us is pure.

Our temptation is to ask them to take control of our awakening, and to be the source of wisdom on our journey. We do this because we think they have access to higher consciousness than ourselves.

This may be true when we first start down our path, because the pipe connecting us to our own source of infinite intelligence can be blocked by pain and density. However, once we attain greater purity and higher levels of connection to our souls, we may be granted access to the same levels of wisdom as these deities, depending on the dimensions that our souls belong to.

I certainly started my journey this way and it served me well, until my connection to my soul was clearer. Eventually, I came to know that my inner wisdom is connected to the same infinite intelligence as every other being in the universe, including the archangels and the great masters, by virtue of the oneness that we share. I now speak directly to my own heart and trust its response, rather than always going to other deities for guidance. It can access whatever I need anytime I like. My metaphysical mentors remain as my friends, and I know they are always present whenever I need their support.

You will know when you arrive at this point of knowing.

Let this be a line in the sand for you. You will become aware of what you are connected to, and what the greatest adventure your heart is urging you to take. You are life living life in full connection to it all. Let it be what it already is. Only you are getting in the way of what is possible, most likely because you have not been fully aware of what is possible, or you fear the truth.

Cross the bridge that can connect you to your truth on the other side of the desert within which you are lost. All that's stopping you from finding your oasis of self-love is the mirage telling you that it does not exist. It's just a story you made up with the assistance of others.

Let the mirage go and enter the natural oasis of love that awaits you!

CHAPTER 5

Your Way, Your Truth, Your Light

Changing the Way We Change

In the Bible, Jesus Christ is reported to have referred to himself as 'the Way, the Truth, and the Light'. I believe that this message has been misinterpreted by many. In fact, he told me so in a channel session that we shared together.

Regardless of your religious persuasions or otherwise, this phrase has a deep significance when we consider the potency of pain, and its role in helping us find our true selves in life. It is an enabler of conscious awareness. Joy can be as well, and that is an even more advanced journey, because responding to joy with change is not a common response.

What Jesus really meant is that, by adopting consciousness in your life and its many experiences, you can tune into your own truth, and ultimately find the light or joy within your own heart. He was not urging us to find his light, but our own light, for we are all a source of eternal love or light.

He had already found his and didn't need our help to do it, because he was already highly evolved when he walked upon the Earth as Jesus!

The word 'way' has a direct correlation to the conscious way of being that is available to us all, once we can comprehend its role in our lives and can do the work to master it. However, in our world, many people live subconsciously because they are yet to master the conscious beliefs within their minds, and to accept that events occur in their life for the purpose of allowing them to grow.

Unfortunately, the way most of us learn is through pain and hard times. I lived this way for much of my life. But until recently I never learned enough from bad experiences. I just tried to change my circumstances without challenging the creator of those painful experience through the attainment of higher consciousness. That creator was me, always.

Like it or not, our lives can be punctuated by disruption, and the ensuing pain that this creates for us. None of us like to 'fail' in our lives, and yet there is truly no such thing in life as failure. All that happens, when we believe we have failed, is that we have not met the expectations that we set for ourselves, or that others set or demanded from us.

We are more likely to learn from a perceived failure than from a resounding success. That is the simply the way most of us operate, because we do not want failure to repeat.

Success, though, can come as often as it wants, for we will always welcome it. As the famous saying goes: *success has a thousand fathers, failure is an orphan.*

Unfortunately, the widely accepted principle inherent in our modern times is that we must regularly set ourselves goals to achieve. This is the mantra of many respected coaches, thought leaders, and business executives.

Expectations can set us up for the illusion of failure, by creating the delusion of what should, could, or would have been if we had behaved differently. Could, would and should are terms, more often than not, derived from the language of our egocentric minds and are best avoided to limit self-deprecation.

An *illusion* is an internal paradigm, which you create yourself and perceive through your sensory perception. A *delusion* is a distorted belief or altered reality that you project to the outside world because of your illusions. They operate in the same way that everything naturally operates in our lives, from the inside out.

Much of the journey to higher consciousness is about dispelling the illusory conditioning that our minds keep us wedded to and mired within. This allows your soul to ultimately merge your human being and light being to become your true human, light being.

But beware, your soul will often smash your illusions to create learning opportunities for you as a human being, and experiences for itself. This can be painful for the human being that you are. We are ultimately life force expressing itself in the physical realm for purpose. When we understand this, we can view our lives as a series of experiences for joy or learning, or both. We are not here to achieve a specific set of material outcomes, or reach a certain destination – how many suitcases have you seen at a funeral? We have choices, and what matters is far more than matter itself.

We do have a divine intent or purpose to our lives that we agreed to before birth. However, discovering this divine destiny, and activating the divinity code within us, is only possible when you remove the density that you are carrying, such that your soul or true self bursts forth from within you. Historically this has been the experience of a miniscule proportion of the population. However, the divine energies that I spoke of earlier, which are now present in our world, are making this state far easier to access.

The concepts of hoping, expecting, needing and assuming are closely related to the fallacy that we can fully control our lives. It is a narrow viewpoint, born from centuries of believing that human beings hold the ultimate intelligence controlling our lives, and that we are separate from universal energies.

This is incorrect.

All are entitled to their views in life, as the Earth is a place of choice and decisions, as I have said.

But fresh perspectives on the way life actually works for us all, has been shared with me through a series of personal interactions with the infinite and loving intelligence to which we are all subject. We need to accept and understand that the universe interacts with our beliefs in an incredible and loving way.

Once we understand this, we can work with it, and not against it.

Resistance can be extremely painful, because if we hold any limiting belief, the universe, through your soul, will eventually bring forth the fear that resides within that belief, to show us that the belief is not valid and needs to be reassessed. This is the universe's way of holding up a mirror to your consciousness, so you can reflect on the new levels of self-awareness that might be possible for you. The universe will do this when it thinks you are ready to deal with the challenges you need to confront. In essence, our fears will often manifest into reality for purpose.

But of course, you are far more likely to receive the lesson that is gifted to you, in a positive way, if you are in tune with the wisdom cascading from the situation. We must work with what unfolds, not what we might hope for or expect in the illusions generated by our minds, so that we can expand our very understanding and knowing of ourselves.

Life is about recognising that we are always where we are meant to be – in the 'isness' of life for purpose. This refers to an ability to accept what is! We can only grow from where we are, not where we hoped to be, like a great oak tree in a forest. In short, bad things always happen for a reason. We can embrace that reality or remain resentful about them occurring. It's a choice.

In effect, we are the centre of our own universe, so knowing ourselves is critical to truly creating the life we want and our 'way' in life.

Evolution sometimes requires contemplation beyond what we have been taught and have become conditioned to believe. Our relative levels of awareness and self-awareness, derived from conscious advancement, are the great differentiators in this world. It ultimately determines how inspiring and fulfilling our lives can become and what we can create.

With that in mind, let's consider the 'way' forward, and its indelible link to pain and the gaining of greater awareness.

Becoming Mired in Misery is Not Your Natural 'Way'

For the first 53 years of my life, I tended to stubbornly stay for too long in situations or relationships that were not positive for me. I found it hard to let them go and look for what needed to change to improve my circumstances. This included employment, friendships, and romantic relationships, just to name a few.

My habit of being too resilient and righteous for my own good meant that sometimes I was determined to win the unwinnable contest. My refusal to fail and accept it blocked me from being fully present and compassionate to the feelings of all involved in each situation, including me.

But, if I couldn't fully access my feelings, what chance did I have of accessing the feelings of others, and fully appreciating the energy between us that needed to be addressed?

As a result, my egoic mind sometimes drove me to persist in circumstances, whereas my happiness demanded that I change my stance. Thus, I struggled to see the virtues of surrendering or compromising in the interests of all. Often the change I needed, but could not accept, was eventually forced upon me by circumstances.

However, this was only after I, and others, had suffered for far too long.

By allowing yourself to really feel into situations, and asking your heart for its loving advice, you can find your way to far more harmonious outcomes for you and others, leading to new paradigms of fulfilment.

This starts with an acknowledgement of the pain that you are most likely suffering from or suppressing, in any given moment.

While we can experience a lot of pain in our lives, we are somewhat unskilled at dealing with it, so it deals with us instead. Because we don't want to get upset or upset others, because as a society we fear emotional outbursts and avoid conflict, we hold our true feelings inside to our own detriment or discuss them behind people's backs with others not even involved. We therefore suppress feelings that arise, and add them to our piles of unprocessed feelings, rather than allow them to be understood, actioned, and released; then continue to judge those who are highly expressive and emotional.

All this leads to negative feelings between people remaining unexpressed, and those feelings getting stuck in perpetuity in the psyches of all those involved. This can be very destructive and block possibilities of forgiveness, reconciliation, and advancement.

The separation between different ethnic races in the world is a prime example of this toxic energy continuing in perpetuity and being passed down through generations. There is so much history of persecution, wars and discrimination, that progress to achieve peaceful reconciliations is extremely slow to evolve and can even get worse over time. Compassion for the plight of the other people and their perspectives is what is needed to achieve harmony; but compassion requires the full accessing of feelings on both sides to be possible. Often this is not an option because our egos are in control, not our hearts, and our egos don't like feelings.

Even a simple rethinking of our previous thoughts requires our minds to admit that it was wrong in the first place, which can be hard to do. But unless we push past this, we can become mired in circumstances or habits of living we may not be truly happy in – the devil you know, so to speak!

Fortunately, there are 'ways' to resolve this.

On the advice of a mentor, I once wrote letters to all the significant people in my life where I felt conflict or tension had not been fully resolved, then visited them to seek a more harmonious outcome on the events that had taken place. This had great outcomes generally, bringing me closer to those people, although there were a minority of people who were not open to the discussion. I could not change what had happened, but in several cases I was able to restate the energy of the events that took place. The expression of my truth, be it too slow in most cases, was a catalyst for enhanced relationships with those with whom I communicated.

The 'Truth' of Life Force

Life is a great privilege. Do you ever stop to think about the miracle that your life is, and therefore by definition what a miracle you are? People will look at a baby after it is born and consider it a miracle, but we were all babies once. Doesn't that make us all miracles?

There are many ways you can live your life. Your options, in a free country like most of the Western world, are quite varied and often open to your desires. But whatever you choose to do, there are certain miraculous truths to consider.

Firstly, you are life force living life. Thus, the life force energy within you will continue to live life through you, if you simply allow it to; and this life force energy is connected to all things, including nature and the rest of the universe. It naturally brings great self-awareness to your being, for it is the only part of you that is truly eternal and has memories and experiences far beyond that of your mind. Your egocentric mind only understands what it has encountered in this life, and in universal terms a human life span is not very long at all.

The intelligence of your soul is infinite. It has extensive memories from eons of years of living as you – your soul energy – and has the ability to access the infinite wisdom in the universal field. Of course, it will not access everything for you, unless you are very highly evolved, only what you need to know to live the life you are meant to live.

So why not surrender to and co-create your life with your inner-sense, for it is your link to the infinite wisdom that you are. And this needs us to feel our way through our lives more.

When you surrender, you are effectively trusting that you are in the arms of the universe, and higher intelligence that loves you. Your soul knows your future. Would you rather trust it to run your life, or an illusory personality that has no idea what your future is meant to be?

True safety lies in your soul, not in the arms of your conditioned mind, and its many illusory and distorted thoughts.

Trust is the cornerstone of all fulfilling relationships. When you trust that you are deserving of a wonderful life, and that your heart knows the essence of your divine plan – and therefore what you need to become to align with it – you are in the right energy to find your way back home to a beautiful and loving life, rich in opportunity.

Resistance is a form of control, and the universe will not co-create positively with a controlling mind. Resist, and what you are currently experiencing will persist, as the great spiritual teachers have professed, and this may result in unpleasant lessons coming into your life for purpose.

In my life, I used to see unhappy experiences as mistakes, or even failures on my behalf. I used to 'beat myself up' and call myself a failure as my perceived mistakes began to aggregate. This ultimately made me untrusting of myself, particularly with respect to romantic relationships. Situations in which my hopes and expectations were not met on numerous occasions left me reluctant to try again. I began to distrust my heart and its ability to discern or lead me into loving opportunities. I blamed the universe for unfairly 'doing me over' and I went into a kind of cocoon because I thought it would keep me safe. But ultimately all it did was make me lonely and unfulfilled.

Eventually, I fell into the truth. My heart led me to the experiences I needed, because they were ladened with the love and learnings I needed to have. However, my egoic and 'safety first' mindset was truly the problem. It had created my pain through its obsession with setting goals and expectations and had always convinced me that others were in fact to blame for any less than ideal circumstances that arose. In effect, I lost trust in myself, and had moved heavily into the energy of control to make sure my life had minimal failures.

Trusting infinite intelligence is always a better option than trusting the limited intelligence of the mind. This is a lesson that I learned the hard way.

The shift from knowledge (originating out of memories accumulated in our minds) to knowing (felt in our bodies and interpreted by our minds) is a powerful one that allows you to trust your heart. However, this shift does not come easily for many, as it is contrary to the normal way we have been taught to live. Knowing must be experienced and felt, and this subtle shift can take a lifetime for some to unfold.

Equally, for some people, it can be instant or come without effort.

This took me years to truly embody this knowing, even after I had understood the principles in my mind from my spiritual research and coaching.

Enlightenment is never an achievement because it can never arise from simply doing. It arises primarily from being and then experiencing something in reality, such that you enter the paradigm of knowing. It is in essence bestowed upon you as you grow your self-awareness. Enlightened ones, like Jesus and Buddha, are renowned for being humble and composed, for they know the truth - that we are all equal and connected to the one source of wisdom.

Your true consciousness is in a different stratosphere to that which your mind can attain. That's why your mind can never attain pure consciousness. It will think it can – but it cannot.

We are all life force, simply experiencing life at different stages on the evolutionary path, a path that never ends. Comparing yourself to others is a recipe for much pain.

The reality is that we are all home in the arms of God. We always were and always will be. Our time on Earth is no more than a kind of school excursion meant to teach us something and be fun at the same time.

But why is the timing of our shift to higher consciousness so unpredictable and mysterious?

The 'Truth' of Higher Consciousness

Our level of consciousness is directly linked to our underlying energies and vibrations.

Our minds and energy fields can carry many limiting energies, which have emerged in this life and/or past or concurrent lives, often referred to as conditioning and/or karma. This is deeply embedded in our subconscious and conscious belief structures and energy fields. It is also mirrored in our bodies, for we are wholistic beings; and it can mask our true level of evolution, which is normally much higher than the vibration we might exhibit or carry into our lives on Earth.

Many of us have been caught in the karmic cycle synonymous with life on Earth, and voluntarily return to restate these karmic energies, lifetime after lifetime. Unfortunately, in the absence of high enough self-awareness we can make these karmic energies even worse. Rising universal energies at this time are, however, challenging us more and more to face our pain, and bringing us the awareness that can assist us to clear our karmic debts.

Our soul vibrations are often very high and may be dimensions higher than the ones we allow ourselves to live within this life. When we incarnate onto the Earth, we are programmed to forget our soul's memories and are placed into unique environments and circumstances in which we can grow further in love. These can be quite harsh but are always chosen by our souls for the benefit of our eternal being. Essentially, the light is exploring the 3D world and using our physical experience for its own evolution. Your body and mind are part of an experiment, in a sense. So why take it too seriously?

This is one of the key reasons we are on this planet and enjoy the great privilege of being alive in the physical realm – so that that our true selves can expand and enjoy the many pleasures and unique possibilities of being in the physical realm.

Our vibration is a spiritual term that could be readily replaced by the word lightness. The lighter we are the higher we are in vibration, for the closer we are to our light. It influences the way we feel about life and respond to it.

It is ultimately possible, therefore, to find our universal connection back to the metaphysical realm while we are still living our three-dimensional experiences on this planet and to embody our full light being. After all, it is your eternal self and the only enduring aspect of you that truly matters in the end, from a universal perspective. So why not do the awareness 'work' to align with the energy of your soul while you are alive and have the adventure it truly wants you to have? It's knocking on the door within you, so why not do the self-awareness 'work' to let it in?

This lightness can be fully gained once the metaphorical holy grail of higher awareness is discovered within you. This is a wisdom mankind has largely forgotten – more on this to come.

This is not a criticism; it is part of the human challenge while we are in form. Our minds and bodies are temporary tools that we are born with and get to use for the duration of our current life on Earth. They are therefore somewhat detached from our universal truths unless we 'do the inner work' to allow all three aspects of ourselves (i.e. mind, body and spirit) to come into wholeness and natural balance.

Our journey back to our truths are, to a large extent, not a learning experience at all, at least not initially; but an un-learning and remembering experience, for to align our hearts and minds we need to effectively allow limiting beliefs in our minds to be exposed and replaced by truths.

Some of these beliefs will be conscious, and some of them will be subconscious. Either way, they are likely holding us back and keeping us trapped in self-deprecating ways of thinking and behaving.

When we unlearn what we have been taught to think in this incarnation and concurrent lives, we open the door for our eternal memories or truths to surface from within us. That's why I used the word 'remember' in the sub-title of this book, rather than a word like 'find'. We are not really seeking something new on our journey to enlightenment, we are opening ourselves up to remember what our universal self already knows, including what it knows of itself. Once you die and return fully in your consciousness to the metaphysical realms, you will become fully aware of all your truths.

When we go through the enlightenment process, we are essentially removing the density we have been carrying in our energies and physical forms from limiting beliefs, or fears. Removing this shadow energy or darkness allows our inherent and eternal light to come shining through, a light that we already are.

This consciousness within us does not need to 'work' on its vibration for it already is at a vibration that is far greater than our minds could ever orchestrate for us. Our role is to remove the debris or density that essentially stops this eternal force from coming through into our Earthly experience in its fullness.

Searching is aligned with the fear-based energy of need. Remembering our truth is a natural gift and it's what your soul wants you to do.

Our souls don't hold such limiting beliefs, so they strive through certain means to bring these limiting beliefs and karmic energies to our attention, so we can release them back into the ether and, in turn, live a more natural life.

The enlightenment process entails shedding, or letting go of, our attachments, karma, limiting beliefs, pains, toxic relationships and negative energies so we can support the emergence of the lighter, brighter soul within us, then allow life to show us what we were truly born to be and do. It takes us back to the child we were originally born to be, free and aware, and ready to explore this planet with curiosity (before the world knocked this out of us). It can therefore take great courage and can be confronting to choose this path back to our truth.

As we evolve into higher consciousness, we eventually learn one big lesson: that we are no-thing. We are not irrelevant, for we are known in both the physical and non-physical realms; but we are the pure energy of love – which is not solid – a no-thing beyond matter. And love is ultimately the source of everything that matters in this universe.

This is an exciting opportunity that many of us are starting to step into out of curiosity, but perhaps without the full understanding of what is possible, and awaits us should we respond in a natural way as life unfolds.

But why should you consider taking this journey of expansion – which can be confronting and even uncomfortable at times? The answer is that it can, and almost certainly will, give you a constantly improving experience of yourself during your life, and end much of the suffering you may have been experiencing and accepting. It does this by changing the way you see your life and by giving you greater wisdom to make your life choices.

It certainly did for me. The shift in my personal paradigm of life brought me so much joy and helped me create a lighter me. However, I admit, it has been difficult at times to get to this point. It has taken a great determination to constantly learn and grow. It has been my choice of course – to remember the eternal truth of me and see how that can inspire me to a better life, more aligned with love.

Eventually, I know I will die and rest in my purity in the metaphysical realms, so why not become that energy before I physically pass on to my next adventure and rest in peace now?

Transforming Into Your Own 'Light'

There are a set of principles that can be applied by any individual to achieve sustainable and inspirational levels of transformation.

These worked for me, and I believe they will work for you!

With guidance from my metaphysical mentors, I have embodied these principles into the Arc, which can build a 'bridge' between you and a better life, between your current experiences and a future that you cannot yet imagine.

Like a rainbow emerging after a storm, the tears you may encounter from opening to your pain combined with the light that will begin to illuminate from within you, will allow this Arc to bring forth greater colour and beauty into your life. New possibilities can't help but shine forth.

The Arc offers you a model you can apply alone if you choose to, or in communion with others. It is a natural process, and you can determine the speed at which you undertake it. After all, your soul knows you have eternity to find your purity if you want it. You might just need a pit-stop at the end to pick up a new vehicle and pit-crew with whom to continue your journey!

It has brought forth a new me that is higher in love, creativity, intelligence, and energy, and largely intolerant of suffering. It has helped me to dream again, like I did when I was a child.

I found this journey astonishing and addictive. It has given me a new lease of life. Let me show you the path less travelled, but one that your heart wants you to consider taking.

Your expansion never ends of course, but it does get easier once you align with the vibration of love and allow your soul to have a greater influence over your life. As you confront your limiting beliefs, fears and validations one by one, they will have a lesser hold over you and gradually diminish in their influence on your life.

Ultimately, your journey to enlightenment will allow you to experience the better integration and balancing of your light being and human being. You are already both, but the human ego normally blocks our awareness of our metaphysical light being, until the ego is sufficiently dissolved by love. In denial and ignorance, the ego creates a kind of veil between the mind and soul, which blocks you from experiencing your full duality in this life. It does this because it does not have the experience of knowing your light being – until it eventually does.

The journey to the light represents a challenging iteration. You go through great highs as your vibration lifts. However, as realisations are felt at different vibrations and within different chakras within you, you can experience perceived density again, as your wholeness processes this density, and the associated beliefs. Even the advanced stages of moving into your light can be challenging, after years of opening to the truth that you are, because the final dissolving of the ego can be extremely challenging. The ego believes it is the source of our awakening, which it can never be. So, the later stages of your journey can interestingly prove to be the hardest, even after all your previous learnings, as the soul moves to effectively dissolve the final remnants of your ego. The Dark Night of the Soul, discussed later in the book, is often a distinct element of this dissolution process.

Once your full integration is felt and known, your consciousness can fundamentally operate in different dimensions simultaneously. You can be in the 3D world with a physical body and brain, yet also access the intelligences of higher dimensions through your metaphysical self. And this access operates at a speed faster than the speed of light itself.

Being fully-filled by your light being will illuminate your body, making you appear to be more radiant or translucent. It will open previously dormant chambers within your brain and enhance your physicality in different ways.

As a result, real fulfilment and new abilities will enter your life. This is your natural state as a human being, and it will allow you to become advanced normality. In other words, you will be able to live in an extraordinary way as an ordinary person, for you will have found the way to your light and your truth.

The vibrations of light upon the Earth are currently lifting and moving more into that of love. The dark ages are well and truly ending. This is making any life lived from the place of ego, highly difficult to endure. For those readers who are sensing this shift and want to move more into the vibrations of what has been termed the New Earth, embracing the journey to your light is one you may not want to miss.

Imagine a world where many people wake up and remove the veils that their egos had previously created to block their light beings from taking control of their lives. This great unveiling is our future, and in fact is already underway for many.

If this sounds interesting to you, why not join this great adventure. It will challenge you greatly, but it's also extremely fascinating.

WE CHOOSE OUR OWN PATH

CHAPTER 6

The Choices We Must Make

Choose Wisely

Now that I have introduced you to the inescapable truth of the metaphysical realm and its universal truths, it's time to acknowledge fully that everything in your life is a choice. Some things we choose before we are born, like who our parents will be, our sex and the body we will inhabit; and some things we choose after we incarnate. Through all these choices, we set a life path for ourselves, designed to challenge us to reach higher levels of consciousness and truth.

The journey to higher conscious awareness requires those who embrace it fully to take full responsibility for their circumstances and lessons. To do otherwise will hold back your expansion and progress towards remembering your divine truths.

Unfortunately, by exercising further choices once we are living our 3D lives, we can often stray further from our intended path out of ignorance – and most of us do.

The Arc can help you rediscover your true self and true path, particularly if you combine it with other practices to stimulate your self-awareness, including certain spiritual modalities. I discuss these options later in this book.

Rediscovering my truth is what happened to me after my life seemingly fell apart in my 50s. The reality is that it didn't fall apart, it fell back into place – finally!

So, the first choice you must make is to read on with an open mind, heart, and hope – because this book is likely to change your whole perspective on life. After all, that is the point of transformation! Transformation is change on steroids, derived from surrendering to whole new paradigms!

I have personally lived through every aspect of this book and applied every concept to transform my own life. There is not one concept I have not put into practice myself.

That said, while I have been coached by learned human and metaphysical beings throughout my journey, and while what I describe in this book has been the greatest experience of my life, I am far from perfect, and much of what I discuss has arisen from opening to my imperfections and the lack of self-love that arose in my mind. Indeed, I have been tested and broken by life many times, to the point where I feared at times that all hope was lost. In this regard, I am very normal and do not hold myself out to be above others in any way.

But with this book, I intend to give you all the secrets I never had when I started my own transformation journey, to help you change the you-that-you-think-you-are, into the you-that-you-really-are.

Why would you want to be anything else but the truest you?

What have you got to lose, except for the real you, who perhaps you've never truly met?

Trust in Love and Accept What is

To allow yourself to be in a place of truth, you must choose to trust and accept that the universe knows exactly *where* you need to be and *what* you need to be, always. You are not alone, even in your darkest moments.

This can be a difficult concept for many to grasp, believing that the universe is the source of your wisdom and wellbeing, particularly when the circumstances of their life get difficult.

We have all had bad things happen to us, and as a result we can often lose trust in life, or resist what is. This is tantamount to losing trust in love, for ultimately *all* is love. But trust, acceptance, truth, and love are all intertwined. In the energy of love, we *can* trust and accept our deepest truths.

I lost trust in love at different points of my life because I felt let down by a series of unfortunate events that happened to me. But I have now learned the truth of these situations and unearthed the unconscious limiting beliefs that I held. None of the challenging events in my life happened to me, they all happened for me and through me, so that I could expand and grow into what I was meant to become.

To apply the Arc effectively, you will need to learn to trust in love and accept that you are always where you are meant to be. To do this, you will need to trust that your own heart knows what is in your best interests. You will need to face your mind's needs, and listen to your heart's wants as a priority. This can be hard to do, but ultimately it is the way we are naturally meant to live – in love, as love, for love.

Surrender to love and you will never look back, other than with great gratitude for what then unfolds in your life. This is where true presence can be discovered and the energy of universal love within you can be remembered and felt.

The Choice is Yours – and Only Yours!

It matters not to me whether you choose to adopt the principles brought forth by this book. But, if you wish to fully embrace the possibilities that await you, you must choose to believe that there is a different way to live your life, to help you deal with hardships, enabling you to come out stronger and wiser. Please don't make this choice because I am advising you to make it. This choice needs to come from your own heart.

It is often said we can turn our greatest weaknesses into our greatest strengths. With this book, you *can* access a tested blueprint to make that inversion a reality now, in every aspect of your life. But it will be up to you to choose to follow that blueprint, and consciously overcome your conditioning, to enable you to become even more conscious.

Conditioning can cause us to stumble blindly through our lives, unknowingly missing our divine opportunities. But that doesn't need to be the case. I am a walking, talking representation of that!

The path to higher consciousness is a journey of discovery that allows us to remember what-we-are and what-we-are-not. Many concepts in this book may be completely new to you; yet, as you read on, you should start to feel like you are remembering them, rather than learning them for the first time. This is because your soul already knows the truths this book teaches, and your soul wants your mind to hear those truths, so you can remember, then become all that you are capable of being.

This is the doorway to true fulfilment, which at present I believe that only a minority of people feel and understand, because they use the surrogates of external recognition and material success to define their happiness. These attributes can help you feel like you are fulfilled, until your circumstances change for the worse, and you are exposed to the highs and lows of life – for purpose of course.

You only see who is vulnerable and 'swimming naked' when the tide goes out. My tide went out a number of times in my life, and this finally awakened me to the cold, hard truths of my reality, and how I was causing every loss and disruption I encountered.

It is your chance to join the advanced minority, to arrive at a higher state of consciousness and to banish pain to your past, such that it no longer impacts your life to any meaningful extent. This advanced principle is well within your grasp, should you choose to be open to it.

We have eternity at our disposal, and consciousness is always expanding naturally; but we can choose to expand ourselves sooner and quicker with advice from those who have walked the path. That is what this book is all about – giving you the awareness to consciously choose your preferred path forward and fully own it as yours.

Prepare to Expand!

The metaphysical truths I espouse in this book burst forth into my life without prompting in 2014.

A series of incredible metaphysical events took place at this time in my life. They were powerful and undeniable. They catapulted me into an advanced new paradigm that dissolved many of my conditioned fears and stoked my ever-present curiosity to new heights.

When people can see and be in contact with life beyond the grave, they no longer consciously fear death or insignificance, because they realise that whatever happens in this life doesn't really matter as much as we think, because they can choose to have another go in their future.

Ironically, as you follow the same path of realisation, you will emerge into a new paradigm where you can trust and love life far more than ever. Your need for external reference points diminishes with higher awareness because, at your very core, you will learn to trust your own intuitive intelligence and the fact that the universe to which you belong is in full support of you.

You will know your heart's desires and you will become more centred within them. Your fears will dissolve, for your true self holds no fears. Your true self possesses the perfection of God, for it is an aspect of God.

As human beings, we are all caught in an ongoing and mighty battle for ascendancy between our perfect and eternal souls on one side, and our temporary minds and bodies that are intrinsically imperfect on the other. This is the great challenge of the human experience, which we can relish with great delight once we become aware of its truth and understand how we can benefit from it.

Higher conscious awareness is a superpower that we all have the capacity to remember. It is not found in the mind. It is found in your true self: your soul. The mind is just the receiver of the wisdom that comes forth from your soul. The mind can hold awareness; but self-awareness can only ever be felt and heard through your body as it is relayed from your soul. It's the mind's natural role to just receive and interpret this wisdom – not to make it up!

As we expand in self-awareness, however, we can explore the world with far more confidence and wisdom. Then, we can use that exploration for further expansion. This cycle of expansion and exploration can go on and on until we leave this planet. But it's so much easier without the suffocating forces of fear, and the pain that it brings forth.

Once you discover this new way of existing and growing, the old ways dissolve, together with the fear and pain life so cleverly uses to bring us into our truth, and back to the fear-less path we are meant to be on – our divine path.

You are not here by chance. There is no chance of that!

CHAPTER 7

My Path Through Pain to Infinite Possibilities

The Awakening Experience

In my book Where Your Happiness Hides, I detailed my initial personal awakening, and how I stumbled onto the path that would eventually transform me and my life for the better. That book discusses the limiting beliefs that so often place a barrier between us and our full potential to awaken.

Awakening is a term often used in spiritual circles, but to me it merely describes the process by which someone starts to comprehend and feel into the who and what they really are, rather than who or what they thought they were. Essentially, a truer story of oneself can start to emerge.

Your awakening is a natural process that will occur for you when you are ready. It is ultimately a matter for you and God. I describe my awakening experience in this book and the natural process I remembered. It helped me to benefit from the amazing events and feelings that were being brought into my conscious awareness to help me expand.

If you are reading this book, you may have experienced an awakening and a call to expand your consciousness. Everyone's awakening is different. Mine was somewhat explosive but I believe it needed to be to shake me free of my entrenched ways of being and thinking. The Arc is my gift to you to assist you in navigating your awakening adventure, no matter how it may unfold.

Nothing in life is perfect, but the circumstances of my own life are far more enthralling now that I can witness them through a more self-aware and awakened lens. The natural journey back to the true self has been an enthralling one for my curious mind.

It began with me finally being brave enough to open to and own my pain, rather than just burying it from the view of others, and to some extent myself. It began with me finally expressing my truth and letting my pain overwhelm me. When I learned to access its messages, and really feel it rather than ignore it, my pain became my greatest teacher.

In a sense, I went from a state of denial to one of destiny.

I only wish that I had been shown this way of being when I was much younger, even in adolescence. I wonder how different my life could have been had my pain and I been friends rather than mortal enemies for all those years. But of course, I know that all is what it is, and I can't change the past, so I am grateful for the awareness that eventually arose and took me under its wing. It helped me to fly to greater levels of peace and happiness.

Expressing my pain retrospectively, and now in real time, has helped me to restate the memories and energetics surrounding past events. I can't change what happened, but I have been able to change the way those events now impact my life and my sense of self. I am proud to say that I have changed the energy I now feel with respect to all the major events in my life. I turned them all from misfortunes into fortunate learning experiences.

I suspect your heart has been whispering these types of secrets to you for years – it just needed a messenger to amplify what it's been trying to bring to your attention. This book is that messenger, offering you truths, and a model to find your own truths, that you can either avoid or embrace. The choice is yours.

My Punctuated Path

The first 53 years of my life were a roller coaster, to say the least. They were punctuated with wonderful periods of perceived success, followed by painful periods of disappointment and loss. To the outside world, I would have appeared to be a relatively successful person with a wonderful family, a strong career, a strong athletic body, high intelligence, and a prosperous lifestyle. I was comfortably well-off compared to many people. But I had several unhappy experiences that left me exasperated and feeling broken.

These experiences included two divorces, the loss of two senior roles (one to illness), the loss of access to my five children at different points, extended family disruptions, and a major muscular disorder that left me physically challenged for nearly 40 years, and seemingly robbed me of much of the pleasures of life that many others seemed to enjoy without the same level of hindrance.

Overall, my life was quite uncomfortable at times, and I suffered from much stress, mental anguish, and low self-esteem.

But, after my second divorce, when my worst nightmares (at that time) came true, I hit rock bottom. I felt completely let down by life. I lost trust in myself.

In hindsight, this was my finest hour – my 'Rubicon' moment, the point at which I could not turn back. I had crossed the river that would allow me to see the source of my pain and eventually love it.

And my pain, combined with my growing self-awareness, were the key architects of the bridge I used to cross that river of discomfort.

It was a profound moment when I turned to open to my pain. I had had enough, and I collapsed into a state of surrender. I had a deep yearning to understand why I had been dealt such awful cards in life, even though I had played with so much good intent, honesty, and energy. I was such a hardworking and committed person, so how could all this damage be done to my life?

My continuous exposure to loss and disruption surely had to have a cause, I felt. And the unspeakable pain I seemed stuck with had to have some purpose.

I felt a driving need to investigate these deep dilemmas with full integrity.

Time and Mentors Did Not Heal Me, I Did

It is often said that time heals all wounds.

My experience has shown that this is not true. It's just a hopeful delusion.

And, of course, time on its own cannot heal any pain that our minds have promulgated within our bodies, through its web of feelings, because our subconscious minds have no connection to time, nor does the reality of karma.

To truly take away this kind of emotionally based pain, we need to work actively to instead dispel the beliefs, or sources of energy, that created the sense of sadness our pain generated in the first place.

Most people only suppress or avoid circumstances that remind them of previously painful experiences. This only serves to divorce them from the opportunities inherent in the circumstances that confronted them.

In this way, it may feel like the problem has gone away; but, unless the person has done the self-exploration and expression necessary to create the required release, the associated pain will still be there and is likely to reappear when similar circumstances arise. Even blaming another person or entity for what took place does not relieve you of the pain; it just allows your mind to artificially discount the pain and put it out of sight and out of mind temporarily. However, it rarely goes away and will reassert itself when certain conditions apply.

For example, you may think you are over a relationship breakdown because you have moved on to a new relationship. But what happens when you come face-to-face with that former partner, who you think betrayed you in the past. In these situations, you will find out how much pain you are still carrying with respect to the separation you endured. It is best to take your learnings from the relationship breakdown, be grateful for those learnings, and forgive all who were involved, including yourself. After all, the breakup represented a great learning opportunity for you, even if you didn't recognise this at the time. However, this forgiveness requires you to face your pain head-on and learn from it.

Forgiveness is a critical element of releasing pain, and it starts with self-forgiveness. Forgiveness is always for the person who holds the pain. If we don't forgive, we can be the custodians of unnecessary pain for the rest of our lives.

For how long do you want to stab yourself with the dagger of pain, when some wise self-reflection could take it away from you forever?

Pain always has purpose, so it rarely goes away without delivering its desired awareness and change. It may come back through different circumstances, or the same ones it once displayed itself from within.

Of course, physical pain can fade as your body heals. Otherwise, pain is just an indicator that something else needs to be addressed, like a flashing light in the cockpit of a plane. It is best to address the flashing lights before you crash, like I did.

Unless we know how to confront and disarm it, emotional pain can feel like a formidable foe.

In my 50s, I found the natural antidote for pain – loving the pain and honouring its presence through expression and exploration, for pain holds the key to removing its own existence. It's like a treasure map: once you find the treasure, the map is no longer of use.

To aid your path to finding greater happiness and enlightenment, I have many real-life examples to share with you about how I found this out for myself. Some of these true stories may be challenging for readers to accept, but I offer them in full authenticity, understanding that each reader can form their own views on what I put forth.

Untruths are not helpful in the search for truth, or along the path to higher conscious awareness.

Meanwhile, your own path to transformation will require commitment and resilience. It is open to all, though it is not for the faint-hearted, or those with a closed mind or heart. It will challenge you to be open to your pain and prepared to look at yourself in the mirror with complete integrity, eyes wide open. It will require you to unlearn beliefs about yourself that you thought were right. It will remind your mind who you really are, after reminding you of what you are not. Time cannot do this for you, it will require you to surrender to what arises and to be prepared to do the inner work on what arose for you.

I have no doubt that my second divorce catapulted me into the journey towards self-love. It felt like the final straw that broke this camel's back. It opened me to truths that astounded me about the real me. It left me with great gratitude for the uncomfortable experiences that befell me, because they lifted the veil I had been wearing, and allowed me to see my true reflection in my own eyes. I held up the mirror and was shocked, but also excited about what I started to see!

What followed my initial detour into intense pain was the opening of my natural understanding of how to expand in consciousness. Once that began, I intuitively followed my instincts, until the detour became a super-highway to higher self-awareness.

That's not to say I didn't have mentors to assist me as my journey unfolded, because I did for years; but there was a part of me that just knew what to do next, like I was remembering it somehow.

In fact, I know I was, and it came from within me, with a little help from my friends!

While you do not need metaphysical mentors to embark on your own journey to enlightenment, and while life mentors here on Earth cannot take the journey for you, I do highly recommend using mentors who you trust, where possible. They will enter your life when you truly need them.

None of us know everything and we can all be guided to our own discoveries quicker with the help of mentors who can spark inner enquiries within us. Each mentor I have encountered on my own path has had different elements of wisdom to share with me and different areas of expertise, and certainly sped up my journey.

My awakening journey is of course never-ending, but it has reached advanced stages much more rapidly because I always respected the input of those more learned than me and, in a discerning way, acted upon their advice.

But still, I had to walk my own path myself – there are no shortcuts.

The key role of evolution is to return us to our pure state of love; that's why the word evolution contains the word love written backwards within it. It has a deeper meaning than we think!

I found it easier to place my attention on my awakening as I got more mature, because I had fewer obligations to tend to and could focus more upon it. It would have been harder in my thirties, when I had five small children and the pressure of making money to provide for my family. So, surprise, surprise, it unfolded at the perfect time!

However, our learnings are always open to us no matter what else we are involved in, or how little time we might have to devote to them. We can always get what we need from every experience we are drawn to, because consciousness is ever present, and it is ready to bring greater awareness through us, for us, whenever we are ready to listen and learn.

Your expansion journey will, therefore, almost certainly be different to mine. They are all unique for we are all unique.

You may be of high evolution already, with your life in a great place. As a result, you may feel no need to expand further through an additional journey to higher self-awareness. I have met some incredibly evolved people who just go about their lives, without seemingly any need for consciousness coaching. Perhaps they are the lucky ones who can find their possibilities without any mentored course correction. Or perhaps they encountered great trauma early in their lives, which led them to course correct themselves and develop a greater self-awareness.

Indeed, many of us only find out how self-aware and secure we truly are when experiencing hard times. We can all be secure and happy when the going is good, but you can only see the rocks on the shore when the tide goes out!

All is a choice and I respect the choices of all. However, no matter how good your life is at present, perhaps there are further possibilities you have not even imagined, which the journey to discovering an even truer you can unveil.

This is an inner exploration, not an outer journey; and no matter how far you choose to venture forth into this adventure, every step you take is valuable, and all matters energetically.

If you have pain or despair, which you have struggled to overcome, venture forth with me into the truths that no one taught you at school or at home, because your parents and teachers were also yet to remember. Come with me to remember what you inherently already know and are opening to in the name of love – YOUR self-love.

It will take time and energy, but it is also a process you will not need to control, for it is a natural state you have just forgotten. I am no messiah, just someone who remembered what life naïvely taught me to forget.

This may feel cryptic at this point, but it will not once I re-mind you of the natural flow that your awakening can bring to your life, that no doubt your soul wants you to embrace with curiosity and intent.

It is time for humanity to see and embrace the gifts that pain can bring to our lives. That way our addiction to suffering can stop.

As we walk our respective paths, we can do so with much more freedom and far less suffering, once we put down the heavy baggage, we all carry in the form of pain and negative energies, which we have never fully released and processed.

There is so much wisdom our hearts are ready to express, through us and for us, when we feel for it, not think it.

This is how the true you can start to emerge. It wants to. It's in your waiting room and ready to take the weight off your shoulders for good!

CHAPTER 8

Preparing For Your Enlightenment

What is Enlightenment?

My original perceptions of the meaning of 'enlightenment' conjured up visions of the Dalai Lama in red robes sitting in a temple, or monks meditating in a monastery high on a hill or sitting in a cave cross-legged. I originally thought that wisdom, once heard, could bring me this thing called enlightenment; which was most likely attained only by sitting with a learned one and absorbing the information and beliefs they possessed, or by reading books that they wrote. In other words, a learning process based on adding to what I understood already.

As my journey unfolded, however, I began to realise that the word 'enlightenment' held the secrets to its own origin, and how to find it.

Consider the prefix 'en'. This relates to something coming from within. Consider the words 'entrance' or 'enjoy'.

And sitting within the word enlightenment is the word 'light'. Of course, when you are light, you are not sad, but happy.

Put the two together and what do you get?

The light – or happiness – coming from within you!

So, enlightenment makes you aware of the happiness and joy you already are. It is not about understanding more than others – it's about BEING light, your light!

You Must Walk the Path

So, if enlightenment is a process of finding the light within you, then it truly does not come from sources outside of you. It can only arrive by tapping into the light that we already possess and applying it in the world we inhabit.

External coaches and mentors can assist us in finding our own light, by steering us through our own reckonings and realisations, but it is only our own experiences of walking our own paths that can take us to enlightenment.

To become the true-you, you can't just think it, you must experience it so you know it; otherwise, enlightenment could easily be gained in a course or book. As an analogy it would be like reading a book on how to play the violin, then thinking you could play one. It takes practice to be able to play the violin proficiently.

We may all dream of being hit by a bolt of lightning, as is depicted in movies, and being instantly transformed into an all-knowing being with super-powers beyond the norm; but unfortunately, this is not how enlightenment works. It must be learned and earned through experiences and embodied to become an integral part of you. You need to eliminate your density of beliefs, energy and form to enable your true self to burst forth from within you. It will not do so until you are of a suitable vibration.

The lessons you are here on Earth to experience, to help you evolve, must be understood and felt through circumstances, so that they can be embodied in your consciousness. Understandings in your mind must become 'knowings' that are also felt in your form.

Once you are enlightened, you will want to apply with great zest the energy that has been awoken inside you. It will be irresistible! You will become activated in ways that only the enlightenment process can unveil. This may change your whole life completely, or just change the way that you feel about and participate in your current life.

In the current energies we are awakening within, you are unlikely to be activated and then sit in a cave or under a tree. Inspiration and action are sure to combine forces for the wellbeing of your life, and that of the world.

But where is our own light and how do we find it?

If you've ever been in a Christian church of any persuasion, you are likely to encounter pictures or statues of Jesus Christ. Typically, he will have a glowing heart and a halo around his head signifying that he is in the light and has a purity the rest of us don't have.

Well, think again, because you are the owner of this same light, you have just not allowed it to surface – yet.

Jesus may be of a higher dimension than your soul, but regardless, your true vibration will most likely be much higher than that which you can currently access in the 3D world.

This will sound like blasphemy to some, particularly to those who grew up worshipping the light of Jesus. *I was one of these souls.* But there is a clear path that can set you on the journey to find your own light. And guess what? This journey will usher you towards far greater enlightenment, if you're not there yet, and most of us are not.

Some people may be there already for various reasons, but they are in the vast minority.

You Will Unleash Your Power

Enlightenment can bring many benefits for those who advance towards it.

When we connect to our light we are connecting to the power of our universal selves. This is in turn connected to our souls. The truth is that this connection has been present all our lives, we have just blocked it through ignorance or pre-conditioned thinking. But it is our natural birthright to know this connection through feeling, just as we did at birth before it was knocked out of us by the traumas and teachings of normal life.

Your soul knows how to activate your full connection to self. Your mind does not. This is why entrusting your awakening to your soul and surrendering to its wisdom is so important on this journey. Your soul has done it all before, in different dimensions and lifetimes. That's why this awakening process is essentially a remembering.

Our universal selves – otherwise called our hearts, because of their link to our heart chakras – possess much greater abilities and powers than our minds, for they have access to our ever-present eternal energy. They are not represented by who we are, by our adopted personality; but by what we are: our true or universal selves, and a source of ever-present energy.

Our personality can best be described as the part of us that believes we are separate from the world and those around us. It is our individual self. It will normally refer to itself in the first person, or as 'I', for it has a separation mindset.

But we are all truly universal. This is our 'U' – the real you, connected to everything and everyone, operating in the universal knowing of unity consciousness, connected to the multiple lives we have lived (or are yet to be conscious of), and the incredible memories accessible far beyond the rudimentary memories of our current minds.

As a result, once we 'clear the pipe' between our true selves and our minds, we can unleash previously unimagined feelings of happiness, psychic powers and levels of intelligence that can literally blow our minds, opening them up to so much more than we currently perceive.

Here lies the real you, not the limited you that you associate with your personality, age, and image.

Can you imagine your true image, or self, coming to light to serve you and the world? And you not needing to buy into or try to be this image and unique self, for it already is you. No effort is required to be your truth because you are it.

Start imagining! For this is where the journey of enlightenment can take you, without needing to become a monk!

Your true self, once rediscovered, will improve your experiences of life, for it is pure creativity, intelligence, awareness, happiness, and love. It will greatly improve your self-esteem because it is the one and only you that is unencumbered by your conditioning and fake beliefs. It is pure self-esteem that you can unleash into your life.

The Beast Becomes the Prince He Already Was

I am often drawn to the 'Beauty and the Beast' fairy story, for it is essentially an enlightenment experience wrapped in a children's story. Many readers will know of it.

As the Beast dissolves his ego and opens to the love he already is, he becomes his true self and discovers true love with the Beauty. The love that he seemingly becomes was there all the time, just waiting to be discovered. He simply had to surrender to it, to remember and feel it. In this process, he became the prince he already was inside his heart.

Perhaps it's time you allowed yourself to look past your imperfections, and open to the perfection of love that lives inside your heart! You don't need a palace to become a prince and to find a beautiful life. It just requires a commitment to expanding your self-awareness, and a willingness to trust in the real you that radiates within.

After all, this is the will of the God within you – the REGENT force you already are!

The Holy Grail is Within Your Grasp

Remembering the truth within you is a wonderful journey, which is why attaining it is regarded as being akin to finding the metaphorical 'holy grail'. The original story of the physical holy grail refers to the cup used by Jesus at the last supper. It was believed to have magical powers, such as the power to heal and provide great abundance to those who possess it.

The legend goes that Sir Galahad, a knight of King Arthur's legendary round table in England, and the son of the great knight Sir Lancelot, was able to find the holy grail with love and peace, unlike his father who had tried and failed to obtain it by force and fear. Clearly this is a metaphor for life!

You have your own holy grail within you – because we all do.

Its powers are also magical and beyond anything you could imagine, although they differ for all of us.

And, just like Sir Galahad, you can find your own holy grail, or light, through the act of loving yourself and then others. The quest to its discovery is guided by love.

Your holy grail is your own heart, and it is ready to radiate its golden beauty into your life, if you let it.

Prepare to Unlearn Who You Are

Consider these snippets of wisdom:

- To be your true somebody, you must first become your true nobody.
- Nothing is the source of everything.
- He or she who needs nothing, gets everything.

These concepts will no doubt represent counter-intuitive concepts to many readers for they contradict many of concepts by which modern man thinks and lives. Mainstream thinking tells us that the way to get what we want in life comes from being of importance, so that we have the money to buy what we want and need. Work hard, take life seriously, self-sacrifice and you will be handsomely rewarded – that is what we are taught from childhood. Essentially, we believe we need to suffer temporarily to achieve our goals in life and find our own version of paradise.

Ultimately, however, we get what we want once we stop needing things. Neediness is based in fear, and therefore its attainments are always temporary from a universal perspective.

Being regarded as important is also a myth. Doing important things matters. Being seen as important does not. We are all important. We don't have to prove it in the eyes of God.

When our egos dissolve, we can become the creator we were always meant to be and create through the endless power of the vibration of love.

So how does all this fit together with the path to greater self-awareness or enlightenment?

We all have conditioned minds – until we don't. To get free of our conditioning requires us to identify those things that make us mistakenly think we are safe and valid. Ultimately, we need none of them, except for the things that sustain and safeguard our physical lives.

Indeed, there is only one place where true belonging and safety lies and that's in our own hearts. When you know deeply who and what you stand for, you can never be lost or feel invalid. You are home and safe in the hands of love.

There is normally only one source of love that you can totally rely upon in this life, and that is your own love. All else is likely to be impacted by egoic conditioning, unless a person you interact with has truly discovered their light.

I found that the initial part of my own awakening process was about what I call 'unlearnings'. This entails exposing your own sources of unnecessary density by:

- *Letting go of past pain and suffering that I was still holding onto.*
- *Releasing any attachment to habits and addictions that were not in my best interests.*
- *Identifying and eliminating things I believed validated my sense of self-worth in life.*

- *Releasing any limiting beliefs that kept me stuck and prevented me from achieving what I was truly capable of.*
- *Freeing myself from toxic and unhealthy relationships, which were not what I really needed and did not really serve my best interests.*
- *Learning to release any new sources of pain that arise as I move through life, quickly and comprehensively, so that pain could not significantly burden my present experiences any longer.*

Any awakening experience can be very satisfying because it creates a lighter and happier you. However, if you approach it with full commitment like I did, it can also be like sitting on an electric fence. Eventually you will want to get off the fence and fully step into the new you that emerges from your learnings. You'll know when this day comes!

Just a word of warning, though: once you achieve a higher level of self-esteem and awareness, from the inner work you have done, you may feel that it's time for a shift in priorities. This may change your life significantly. But the expansion process never fully ends, it just morphs and develops. As you attain new understandings, you will truly grow, once they are embodied into the reality of your 3D experiences.

As you walk your path, clutching the power of the Arc, you may liken yourself to a butterfly, emerging from its chrysalis and fresh from amazing transformations. Initially these transformations will not be visible to others, until you burst forth into the full light of day and fly.

Your inner and outer radiance is likely to amaze those who witness this new you and see you take flight. Your new radiance may confuse others who are witnessing it in you for the first time and can't quite understand how it has arisen.

Such lightness is gained from having less density of thought and feeling. The negative energies we carry through life are linked to beliefs and illusions in our minds, which can manifest as feeling confused about our lives, and be reflected in our energy fields and bodies. They are the source of our limitations and stress; so, if we can unlearn and release them, we can release ourselves from the cages of your own making (I called this the cage of conditioning in my book *Where Your Happiness Hides*).

This unlearning or shedding process must take place before we can start to learn who and what we really are.

We need to let go of our illusions before we can let in our truths.

Love is Nothing and Everything

The above reference to being *nobody* and becoming *nothing* refers to the journey out of ego and into the purity of your own heart. In this way, the enlightenment process is essentially a purification process, for you cannot touch love, it can only ever be felt. It is just energy; no more no less.

Love is thus 'no-thing', and since the universe was created from nothing and *all* is nothing before it becomes something, if we believe in and embody the pure love that you already are, all will be possible for you.

We are ourselves no-things, for we are the eternal vibration of love, connected for eternity to the light of the cosmos.

This, as I said above, does not make us a nobody, as we are known in the physical and metaphysical realms. However, we are essentially light expressing itself on Earth for purpose. Allowing our egos to dissolve, however, allows us to become our true somebodies. The authentic us.

Many of us devote vast amounts of energy in life to making money, developing an attractive image, avoiding pain, and ensuring the world values us, even if we don't value ourselves. People often talk of the desire to find their calling or purpose in life; their minds seek to understand and put a name to this thought.

But the path to enlightenment is paved only in love, and our true calling or purpose in life is born out of love for and in devotion to ourselves. It must be known *and* felt before it can be understood and put into action.

The first step to finding our deeper purpose is self-love; a state that allows you to realise you are pure love, and that we are here on Earth at the behest of a universal love that wants us to love the life we have and the life force that we are. To merely *think* purpose, without feeling and being it through learning to be our true loving selves, is a misnomer that can only result in a concept, more like a job description or mission statement. *Thinking* about your purpose might be fun, but it has limited value, because our minds can never determine our true divine purpose until our souls make it known to our minds.

We all want to love and be loved by others. In the energy of love, however, you can even establish true love with others by merging your love to theirs in a blended field of bliss. We are more powerful than we give ourselves credit for, even in our love lives, because our true selves are supported by the unlimited potential that emanates from love.

I am so grateful that I allowed my soul to show me more of what and who I really am. Now that I know and can feel into the energy that I am, it would be torture for me to go back to the smaller person I once thought I was before. And to be in a romantic relationship with another that is not based on truth and love is no longer tenable for me.

To find your own energy of love, a key step will be to address the energy of fear found in your ego-centric mind. While love has the power of expansion, fear possesses the power of inflation and deflation. When we expand our thoughts through love we become more; whereas when we inflate or deflate our thoughts through fear, we often find ourselves needing more, and never truly growing. We inflate or deflate through need. We expand and grow through want.

The love-that-we-are, our souls, our true selves, dearly want us to expand back to our natural state, to become what we were intended to be; for this love is ever-present, always energised, and knows why you chose to live this life as you, now. It even knows who the people with whom you are intended to experience significant relationships are and decides when you leave this planet. You will not die without its blessing! It loves you unconditionally, for it is the real you. And, even if you deny its presence in your current life, it frankly does not care, because it knows it has eternity to evolve with the different versions of you that arise, so it will never judge you harshly.

To lose all fear in your life ultimately requires you to accept that you are an eternal being with a never-ending energy or life-force that loves you totally. In this place, or paradigm, death becomes less relevant because it is ultimately a redundant concept at a universal level. Death simply opens the door for you to be reborn into a new life. This concept is a hard one to get your mind around for good reason. Your mind knows it will cease to exist once this incarnation ends, for it, like your body, is temporary.

Obviously, none of us want to die in this life, but we must accept its inevitability and possibilities. Death is hard for the human being to accept, but easy for the light being to embrace, because it's done it hundreds of times. It is therefore important for the human being to grieve death and other significant losses, as they arise in our periphery.

If you can progressively dismiss your fears, you can then embark on the journey to finding your divine presence and, once found, discover your divine path – which only your heart knows. It is like the usher in a movie theatre with a torch, always ready to show us where we need to go next, particularly in the darkness.

Awakening is Not Really Healing

Some speak of the awakening process as healing, but this is, to some extent, a falsehood. Deep within us sits pure love, within a pure heart, with full access to infinite intelligence. So, we are the only thing blocking what-we-already-are from coming forth. We are limited by the junk we hold onto and our own limiting beliefs.

The term 'healing' can therefore only refer to the removal of our egoic illusions, and the associated pain and suffering it creates for us, without our conscious knowing.

The term 'healing' infers that something needs to be fixed. But since we are already complete at our core, we just need to get out of the way of our own purity, so that it can be who and what we already are.

This is why, rather than enlightenment 'healing' us, I prefer to refer to the process as a 'remembering'. It is essentially a purification process that allows your full light to come forth from the density that once blocked its emergence. You are remembering your purity.

Key Insights That Await

As you journey progresses closer and closer to higher consciousness, you will have the opportunity to gain a greater understanding of the key insights listed below. When I'm sharing my insights with others, I often find it helpful to state certain concepts upfront, so they can more clearly see and anticipate the path ahead. We have already touched on some of these.

- We can work with the physical and metaphysical aspects of ourselves to grow and expand, for we exist in both.
- Your true self exists independently of your mind, and it is possible to allow the real you to emerge from within all the diversions we are distracted by in our busy lives.
- You *can* transcend the limiting beliefs, behaviours, and fears in your life.
- It is possible for a human being on Earth to commit to a higher level of self-awareness.
- The true powers we all possess, and what you are capable of being, if you are in full connection to your wholeness, has been largely lost and suppressed over the centuries.

- Being highly self-aware gives you a greater opportunity to define what constitute fulfilment and happiness in your life and greater power to manifest it in your reality. This can help you discover the unconditional love that we all truly are and can express with others and with ourselves.
- Karma from this and past lives can be overcome, should you choose to address it in your life.
- Unlearning is more important than learning on the path to enlightenment. As you move closer to the vibration of love in your life, by unlearning who you thought you were, you will effectively release the illusions that kept you trapped in false paradigms of happiness. This unlearning process releases unnecessary density and allows your light being or higher self to fully burst forth into your life.
- The universe constantly works *through* you, and *for* you, to help you expand. Contrary to our normal beliefs, nothing happens *to* you. There is great freedom in this knowing, for it releases the concept of blame from your way of living.
- Pain can bring wisdom to your life, and it has a natural role in our discovery of happiness. Avoiding it is to avoid truth. Loving it and its wisdom is a key step to embracing your reality. Pain is the cousin of joy.
- There is a natural process that we can apply to any difficult experience, to both recover and enjoy a better life. This is the Arc.
- Using the Arc can lead you to higher levels of consciousness.
- Being nothing, and dissolving your ego in the petri dish of love, is one of the most powerful pathways to manifesting your version of true fulfilment and sovereignty, for love is the most potent energy of creation when we allow it to cultivate our lives in an unfettered way. Your light or essence springs forth from a base of love.
- Your beliefs may cause damage to your life, whereas they could be making you a superstar!

- Your egoic mind can never be the source of enlightenment. It will think it is. Therefore, it is important in your awakening process to hand-over your journey to your soul. This is difficult because your mind has got through life thus far and does not want to let go of the reins. But it must eventually relinquish this role and surrender, for you to merge with your light.

Key Principles to Feel Into

There are also some key principles that, once embraced, can make your journey much more effective and enjoyable:

- Change, and on a bigger scale transformation, will need to be embraced even if you feel exposed and 'naked' in the absence of control and certainty. Protecting yourself from change will almost certainly keep you away from the new possibilities that the journey to your truth will bring forth. You must allow the tide to go out and expose your truths. Swim naked!

- Forgiveness. As you progress and open yourself up to your pain and unpleasant events from your past, you will need to forgive yourself and others for their role in your learning opportunities. Blame and shame are the enemies of new learnings and beginnings; they keep you mired and wallowing in the past. They also belie the reality that everything in life has been chosen by you and happens for your benefit – EVERYTHING.

- Valuing new areas of wisdom, and knowing, may not immediately convert into external opportunities or pay-backs. Your inner reality can't help but eventually change your outer reality, if you choose to allow it to do so, once you step into new opportunities and convert your new energies into real outcomes. Wisdom can create wealth, but wealth will never create wisdom!

- The process enunciated in this book is a journey into your own self-love. You are not doing this for others, although they may ultimately benefit from the work you do on yourself. You are living your life for you, not for others. As a result, some people may be critical of your more advanced understandings and learnings. From my experience, it's best to primarily share your experiences with those who are supportive. Match your audience with your disclosures, but never be inauthentic with what you say.

- Love the journey, and in return it will love you back for the rest of your life. The path to higher intelligence is like discovering a genie in a bottle. The returns can be incredible, and once you have attained greater self-awareness you will never fit the genie back into the old bottle. Awareness never goes backwards once attained.

- Confusion always precedes clarity. *I was once confused in my life and constantly seeking peace through certainty. I always wanted to know my future and to plan for it. Ironically, this need for certainty contributed significantly to my confusion and anxiety. Eventually, I learned that my confusion was a gift, as was its associated pain, because it gave me a platform to explore further positive change. I now love confusion when it arises. It peaks my sense of curiosity and sets me on a new enquiry that I know I will learn from, always!*

- Expect the unexpected. My journey brought me into direct contact with the metaphysical realm in many wonderful ways. Who knows what yours will bring forth!

CHAPTER 9

The Battle Between Ego and Soul Energy

Banishing the Ego

Ultimately our egos are our greatest enemies in our quest for our true selves. To be the truth of ourselves, our egos must be dissolved into a greater sense of wholeness, integrating all parts of ourselves: mind, body, soul, and energy into one.

Like a disprin dissolved in water, our egos can and *should* become invisible in our lives. Once we are cleansed of all egoic attachments and validations, and we begin functioning in the energy of the heart, the ego can become less prominent, and only applied in situations when you need to project a certain personality.

You can then dial your adopted personality up or down as needed, but it is temporary, because you know that you are neither needing to project or protect an image to feel whole. Some speak of a person having a healthy ego. However, I prefer to call it an optional ego, as it is one you can use when you need it, then put it back in the draw until you need it again. You own it; it does not own you.

You will still have a functioning mind operating in its natural role as the organiser and interpreter of your heart's desires. However, the mind knows this is not the real and complete you. It is a temporary servant of love, until the day you die.

I had a powerful ego for much of my life and it led me to much suffering. I am still far from perfect, but opening to my pain and ego-based attachments has improved my perspectives on life and my self-esteem.

I spent much of my life trying to avoid the pain of failure or loss. I did this with a controlling mind. But life caught up with me and the universe showed me, in no uncertain terms, where I was in fear. My fears came true because this is how vibration operates in life. Eventually you will always get what you fear. The pain that arose was, however, the gateway to my redemption and a fresh start.

Letting Go Requires Allowing

One of the hardest things to do when we take on the journey to becoming our true selves, is that we often allow the egoic mind to try and control the process. Our souls are the only source of pure consciousness, but our egoic minds like to think *they* are.

I struggled in my own awakening with the application of allowing or surrendering, as do many people with strong controlling minds, like I had for most of my life.

We grow up being taught to *think* our way through life. In places like school and many workplaces, we are rewarded for thinking, not feeling. Logic is seen as our most powerful tool.

Our self-awareness or intuition is our *true* super-power, not that our egos can willingly allow that idea to flourish.

This is because the role of our ego is to protect us and project us to the world for our benefit. It does not like to be subrogated to the soul, as it prefers to think it is not only in-charge of our journey to higher consciousness, but also the source of our consciousness.

This is a subconscious falsehood, though taking this mantle away from the mind can be a great challenge, because our minds will likely have effectively suppressed our feelings and the passion in our hearts for many years. It's therefore extremely difficult to alter any belief that our minds have created, partly because they are often subconscious and therefore not easy to identify, but also because our minds don't like being put out of a job – a job they think they have become highly adept at and believe is theirs for life.

If we try and change our mindsets, without the clarity provided by feelings, our minds may alter the wrong belief or replace it with an equally inappropriate one. Our minds are useful servants along the path to enlightenment, but they cannot control something that is ultimately beyond their comprehension. They are *not* the source of our light. In most cases they are the source of our darkness. But as is often said, we do need darkness to see the light! The battle between your heart and mind is the struggle that needs to be opened to, to take yourself to higher consciousness. This is a major aspect of the human experiment and therefore where great opportunity resides.

Our minds are largely a library of what is already understood. They are great storers of information and memories, but not normally capable of being the originators of new paradigms or possibilities, which forms the basis of personal transformation.

Our souls know what energies we carry and what's in our best interests to release, and when. When given this role, they will apply their unlimited universal wisdom to take us to our truth in divine timing. This timing, which works off the coalescing of energy, will always be in alignment with our true destiny.

When we let our minds control this process, they will try to base it on the timing of the clock and calendar. It will become a process of time frames, deadlines, and expectations; whereas it is a natural process that cares not for our human concept of time, but for the movement of energy and light.

When you start to apply the Arc, or your own version of it, you are consciously entering the realm of quantum physics. This has been documented by other authors, but science is still in the early stages of coming to terms with it. But you need not understand it to adopt it. Your soul has a master's 'degree' in it. You just need to accept its reality and marvel in its incredible power, for it is your natural state to do so and to be supported by it.

I bought into the illusion that my mind could control my awakening multiple times during my journey to higher consciousness before I felt the errors of my ways. I was obsessed, at different points, with my so-called spiritual achievements and the time it took me to get them. But making these mistakes taught me much and now I bring them to you so that you can avoid the mistakes I made!

The wholistic nature of my own reality – the balance and combinations of the energies of our hearts, bodies, and minds – certainly became much clearer as I progressed along my journey, and I began to work with the different aspects of my wholeness simultaneously. The role of my mind in this gradually shifted from one of control and driver, to one of assistant or facilitator of the process. It remained important, but my self-awareness wanted to teach me that my mind was not the source of my self-awareness.

But how do we come up with new ways of being and acting, and bring them forth into our lives? You simply need to be open to receiving them, to silence your mind and ALLOW natural enlightenment happenings to unfold through you, for you. Most tend to occur when you are not trying to create them, because your soul, not your mind, has brought them forth for your benefit.

I experienced my initial awakening when I was simply watching television alone late one night – I had a powerful metaphysical experience that lasted for over an hour. Every light in the house started flashing, and a presence came upon me that felt profoundly pure. Electrical devices, like television sets in different rooms, started turning on and off unexpectantly. The experience was intense, yet I felt completely at peace. It was beautiful and magical. I loved every second of it, even though it felt like I was in the scene of a ghost movie.

From that moment, many other metaphysical events have unfolded around me, including visitations from Archangels Michael and Metatron, and Jesus Christ.

These events aroused my interest in the metaphysical, and initiated my quest to understand what was taking place. Spiritual books and mentors soon began to open my eyes to what was possible when we surrender to the love within us. Much has unfolded since of its own accord. More accurately, I know it occurred at the behest of my soul.

I know that the stress of my second divorce, and the subsequent self-reflection process I undertook to release my pain and expand, unleashed these amazing experiences and the many others that followed. I believe it was an incredible gift to me for opening up to my pain with full integrity.

But more than that, it showed me beyond any reasonable doubt that I was present in duality. I was physical and metaphysical at the same time, and needed to honour this truth and harness it for my wellbeing.

Along your own journey to greater awareness, your soul will also know what *you* need. Even if your path may at times seem more challenging than others, the trick is to trust that your soul knows you and will give you what you need. Your role is to interact with any challenges that arise for you, and through you, so that you can 'establish' a greater connection to yourself – to your real or universal self. This connection already exists. It's truly about you knowing and experiencing this reality.

As issues arise, it is important to feel beneath any pain you experience and allow the love in your heart to help you release it, through the gift of higher self-awareness.

The universe will only ever give you the challenges that you are ready to take on and grow through. So, in effect, the tougher the situations you encounter, the more evolved you are likely to be.

You can't control life's happenings fully anyway, although almost certainly your mind will try to do so – it will not want to give up its throne without a fight, and you will need to be prepared for this, but not self-critical, for it is quite a normal experience to resist this reality when it arises.

Only *you* can help your mind to abdicate its illusory role as the source of your truth and destiny, by surrendering to the love within you and the pain you may be feeling. The true regent is ready to arise!

May the Letting-In Begin

Our journey to higher consciousness is initially comprised of the unlearning process mentioned above. Once we clear away our mental distortions, our personal energy shifts, and the life we are presently living comes into clearer focus, enlightenment can begin to unfold in a far more graceful way.

With our souls in charge, a form of alchemy can begin within us. Our souls begin to redefine the way our minds and bodies operate. There is a new force controlling our lives. And it is far more conscious and powerful than the energy our minds believed they had. This is the way an advanced human being lives. This is the future of life on Earth, with all of us now having greater access to higher dimensional energies, should we choose to 'do the work' to consciously align with them. The veil we subconsciously impose between ourselves, and these energies are now easier to remove, through higher conscious awareness.

When we are born, we already know how to eat, breathe and use our eyes. Our subconscious minds control our body temperature, and our bodies can heal any cut or abrasion we may sustain.

But our souls can do so much more than this, if we allow ourselves to live from love. We can be shown who and what we really are, by the only force that really knows us fully: our souls. There is no more guesswork required, for we can become our true light, and that light can begin to show us our possibilities, not old certainties residing in our repeating patterns of conditioning. We then move from the pain of our current probability to possibility and new paradigms we could never previously imagine. Pain gives way to possibility.

This is often shown to us through inspirational feelings in our bodies and clear whispers that tell us what we would love to do and be a part of. Once we reach this point our role is to listen and step into what we hear and feel. This is the genesis of real passion, not the passion that we think we understand, and which is driven by our conditioned thoughts, and the occasional foray into our hearts.

Messages of knowing can be so much more inspiring, depending on your vibrational and listening capabilities – or in other words, how connected you are to your true self and how much you listen to its knowing and inspirational messages.

The process of knowing thyself is your evolutionary destiny. The higher your vibration rises the more you will discover about yourself. We will all get there when we are ready to do so, when we allow ourselves to stop being inhabited by unaware habits, and to allow our true selves to step forward.

This Arc gives you a natural way to do this.

You are More Than You Think

The path to higher consciousness will require you to work with different aspects of you to different degrees. These aspects can naturally interact with each other every day of your life. The consciousness journey allows you to be mindful of how these different aspects interact, as you start to work with them.

In simple terms, you are comprised of the following four aspects:

1. Your mind, which operates inside your brain.
2. Your body, of which you are acutely aware.
3. Your heart, which is your centre of love and feeling, and which, through the heart chakra, connects you to universal energies and the full power of your soul. This is your eternal home.
4. Your human energy fields.

Your energy field sits around your body and is an electromagnetic source of energy that takes the shape of a luminous egg-shaped object. The human energy field has multiple layers and extends about five metres on all sides of our bodies.

Our fields allow energy flows to traverse to and from the universe, mirror our very being and holds the key to our karma, emotions, mental, spiritual, and physical states. Every field on the planet is different because we are all unique.

Our fields interact directly with our cellular structures as the cells in our bodies mirror and are influenced by our field. This means every time our fields change, we need to integrate the changes into our cellular structure. This can take a few days, and its speed and symptoms vary person by person. This process is natural – your mind can assist it but not control it.

In my case, this process starts instantly and takes about three to five days to feel complete.

The human energy field is complex and plays a vital role in our role to higher awareness. However, from my experience involvement with the human field is largely automatic. You can and will influence it as you evolve, but directly working with it is an advanced aspect of the path to consciousness that can come down the track if you choose it, **like I have**.

It may be time to shed the personality you once knew and unlearn your way to what has always been true. The truth of you has been sitting in the shadows, and is ready to illuminate your way forward. You are naturally radiant, despite what you may have come to believe.

PAIN IS INEVITABLE

CHAPTER 10

How Pain is Misunderstood

The Truth of Pain

Our world is in a constant state of flux – with eight billion souls living on this planet, it can't help but shift on an ongoing basis. The truth is that this never-ending process of change is aligned with the natural order of evolution. We are truly all experiencing what we are meant to experience. We are all here on Earth to expand, just like the universe that holds us.

Energy is always dynamic and moving. It can never stand still. And all is ultimately energy.

By expanding, growing, and interacting with each other, and the various elements of Mother Nature and the galaxy of which we are a part, we must inevitably encounter change, taking place in both our individual lives and as collectives, and change is often a painful experience.

Pain is thus inevitable. Unless you hide under a rock, you probably can't escape it. Change is often described as a constant in our lives. It is natural.

However, mankind has become accustomed to trying to avoid change, unless it's likely to be positive. Our rudimentary minds think that disruption, or change, is something best avoided, for it can bring a healthy dose of pain to our often routine and controlled lives.

Our conditioned minds usually seek safety and security, before they seek adventure. This is the security centre of consciousness, and it influences our NORMAL approach to dealing with disruption and pain. But there is a far more NATURAL way of embracing theses forces in our lives.

Pain is actually the indicator we need to embrace, for it is the intelligent gateway to ultimately living a life substantially free of this often-unwanted guest. It appears in your life for a reason – it wants you to remove it, through higher self-awareness.

Pain is ultimately a loving message from your body and/or soul that you need to change in some way. If you don't listen to it, it is likely to persist because it loves you. It wants you to listen to it and honour its presence with conscious choices.

Pain is natural for humans, and it can be terrible. However, it can also be a great asset in certain circumstances. The bottom line is that nature gave us pain and the intelligence to confront it for a reason.

I have loved mine to create a better life. The ability to feel and express pain, or joy for that matter, is a wonderful trait of being human. It helps us to be real and vulnerable.

When pain is no longer seen as a barrier in the way of joy and happiness, you can pass through it and beyond it, and be grateful that it graced you with its presence and met you in its rawness.

It is a misunderstood gift of nature in many cases.

I recognise that there are different kinds of pain that also have different sources. The primary pain I focus on in this book is the pain that stems from our emotional reactions to life or even past lives. Some might call this stress or self- created negative energies. Stress can have its genesis in the way we react to the circumstances of our life or what we believe, and this can manifest into our physical realities as real bodily pain and distortions.

I describe my personal relationship with this kind of pain later in the book. This is the form of pain that I am directly familiar with and can comment on with authority.

My recurring references to pain in this book are directed at this kind of situation or circumstances. There is of course, physical pain that may arise from unfortunate circumstances that take place in our lives, like accidents, conflicts, and genetic deformities, or even diseases that we could not have foreseen or controlled. People with these forms of pain have my greatest compassion and I am not readily able to pass judgement on these forms of adversity. I will leave this pain to the highly skilled doctors, surgeons and physicians who give people hope and relief.

My only caveat is that I believe all that happens to us in our lives has purpose. We choose everything we encounter. Therefore, all pain has been chosen by our souls for our expansion in some way. However, this is cold comfort to someone who is suffering significantly and has no tangible avenue to ever escape that pain, other than perhaps through drugs or death. As someone who experienced the nightmare of recurring physical pain for many years, I offer my sympathies, because I know how emotionally hard and debilitating this can be.

The Present Paradigm of Pain

For many people, the mere thought of pain conjures up negative emotions and perceptions.

From the moment we are born and taken home with our new families, we are conditioned not to express emotional pain, for instance by crying. Positive expression is valued and encouraged, but not any negative forms of expression. The first hint of crying by an infant or older child is so often met by frantic parental attempts to stop any signs of perceived suffering. Tears and screams are met by differing strategies, to stop them from dominating the environment within which they are heard.

We don't want to sit near crying babies on a plane or endure them in the shopping centre. Crying children must be quickly pacified, or embarrassed parents will go into apology mode. In most cases, the child is crying because it wants attention. However, the child soon learns that its crying is not an acceptable behaviour, and much effort is expended by its carers to curtail the noise and emotions, lest they disturb others or the parents themselves.

As we grow to adulthood, this lack of acceptance of our desire to cry and express negative emotions is deeply established in our psyche. We learn that crying occurs in moments of unhappiness or pain, and therefore, by the time we become adults the patterns are clear: expressing strong negative emotions is to be avoided, particularly in front of others. It's safer to hide and suppress any pain we feel, rather than showing others that we need emotional support, or other forms of aid.

This has historically been heightened in the behaviour of males, because males in many cultures are so often valued for their ability to be stoic, strong, and in control of their emotions. Warriors don't cry!

Crying women are more likely to be tolerated and supported by society, yet in some environments – such as the business circles, in which I spent nearly 40 years – a crying woman is often deemed to be lacking resilience and the power to compete. Cry and she is quickly relegated below the status of those who don't, or who hide the fact that they want to or do in private.

Pain itself can arise from many different experiences. It can be derived from unwanted physical outcomes relating to accidents or diseases, remorse relating to death or morbidity, relationship breakdowns, loss of wealth or employment, or threats to your safety and security. This list is long because pain is intrinsic in our makeup as human beings. But whatever the type of pain experienced, we tend to believe that expressing pain in front of others will make us appear and feel lesser.

But why did nature give us an ability to feel and express pain, if we were supposed to shut down this important sensation within us? What's the point of it? Why hasn't evolution struck it from our repertoire, after all isn't nature supposed to support the survival of the fittest? And surely the stronger and fittest among us are in control of our emotions?

The answer is that many of us have lost the plot when it comes to understanding the critical stories and messages that pain can bring to our consciousness. Pain, and its associated emotions, are cornerstones of the natural processes that can both enlighten us and expand our horizons in life. They are indicators that change of some kind is needed for us to restore our natural equilibrium within. We have lost touch with this powerful tool within us.

But we can learn to face it, listen to it, and use it to our advantage.

Pain as the Purifier

My life and well-being improved dramatically once I learned to open to my pain, to listen to its wisdom, and to love it as a critical part of me. I finally welcomed it into my life. I only wish I had learned to let my pain be my mentor and ally earlier in my life. I am sure I would have had a far better and more enjoyable experience!

But it took me years to face and express the pain that had accumulated over the course of my life, to that point. Of course, this was better late than never in every respect. Taking full responsibility for my pain, both physical and emotional, opened a doorway to a life that I was previously unable to perceive.

With every tear and every release, my pain took me one step closer to my true self and a joy I never knew I could know. It gave me what I needed in my moment of need.

My disease was part of my evolutionary journey and a divine challenge I chose to face before I was born.

My journey has been a wonderful experience, and I am now excited and inspired to share it with you.

Pain is our teacher if we dare to attend its classes and listen to its wisdom. Doing so can help us to hear and become aligned with the harmonics and vibrations that our souls have long been playing within us.

If we can tune into our pain and respect the songs it is playing for us, these chords of seeming discontent can become a conduit for intelligent creation to express itself through us and for us, with beautiful and harmonious outcomes.

When we encounter pain, we may be encouraged by modern medical practitioners to take drugs to suppress its impact on our lives. We may look in the direction of recreational substances, like alcohol or drugs, to mask our negative sensations. Some of us may even be so overwhelmed we consider ending our own lives or seeking revenge on another. Our level of tolerance to pain can vary, and this is quite normal.

However, we need to give due attention and expression to every vibration of pain that our senses detect. Ignoring them can bring great peril to our lives. It is just another form of energy we can release; though not through violence.

There is much violence in our society, including domestic violence. Is this because we have lost our ability to cope with loss and rejection? Are we unskilled at learning from the pain we feel and changing ourselves to ensure we evolve from its presence? Is our expectation that men need to suppress their pain and not express it, leading to women becoming a constant target of pent-up anxieties and insecurities?

Pain is a confidant we can learn to lean upon, and a mentor who allows us to step through great learnings and un-learnings. Our path to purity and possibility is lit up in the presence of pain, like great sunlight striking forth at sunrise. It is the illuminator in our hearts of new beginnings, if we care to honour its natural intentions, and the light that it can bring forth for our benefit through higher awareness.

The 'spiritual' awakening process, as it is commonly referred to, can often feel like a chore in its initial phases. Like finding yourself in a jungle, you may need to hack through dense undergrowth with a big machete to find a river or clearing more to your liking. When you're tackling that undergrowth, it may seem hard or uncomfortable at times. But once you face whatever you need to face in that jungle, you get to relax in a natural place of sheer beauty and comfort.

The truth is, deferring or masking pain is not a great strategy, as I learned the hard way. If we refuse to face it earlier in our lives, when it initially graces us with its presence, we often find ourselves having to face it later, when doing so might be even more inconvenient. And, if we allow ourselves to endure and accumulate pain over time, it will only accumulate and hurt us more than was ever necessary or intended by life. This is no coincidence because the infinite intelligence of the universe inside us brings our lessons forward when it knows we can benefit from them.

The journey through and beyond pain is worth every moment of the commitment that it entails. Its benefits are profound, and the peace awaiting you on the other side is impossible to attain in a sustainable way by suppressing it or trying to go around it with denial, addictions, or substances.

The energy of pain is natural, and only its return to nature, by allowing its energy to be in motion and understood, can ever give you what your heart truly desires – peace and freedom from suffering.

Pain won't kill you because it's just a feeling, but ignoring its wisdom might.

It is time we embraced a different paradigm when it comes to pain and suffering. Come with me on this wonderful journey, seek out the holy grail that will eliminate suffering and pain from your life, and cross the fine line between personal power, pleasure, and pain.

I promise you, you won't regret stepping into this new paradigm!

HOW TO MAKE USE OF PAIN

CHAPTER 11

The Normal Way We Deal With Pain

The Rickety Bridge We Try to Cross

The normal way we try to deal with pain is counterproductive. Let me illustrate this with my own key experiences.

As I mentioned earlier, I lived a sometimes challenging and painful life over my initial 53 years. Yes, the pain I experienced was often offset by periods of great 'successes'; but without a doubt the worries from my past seemed to trump the wonders I experienced.

My greatest problem on this roller-coaster ride was that I did not comprehend the power I could attain by opening to my problems, learning from them in a place of full surrender, and making substantial changes to my beliefs.

Such is the mindset of the perfectionist that I was conditioned to be! Suppress your pain, suck it up, dust yourself off and keep going were my adopted mantras. Don't let people think you can't cope with adversity.

As the British Prime Minister Winston Churchill said during World War II, to enhance the resilience of the English population, "When you are going through hell, just keep going."

Sound familiar?

Of course, herein was the core issue. Instead of completely feeling my pain and owning it, expressing my emotions and experiences and making suitable changes to my life, I instead accumulated a wealth of pain and self-destructive beliefs, none of which I had processed or learned from. They were buried deep inside me and were wreaking havoc on my well-being. They had a powerful influence on my actions and thoughts, and ultimately kept me trapped in a repeating pattern of less-than-ideal outcomes.

I was too intent on appearing to be happy and successful. If other people thought I was a success that was what mattered to me; my precious outward image!

Inwardly, though, my life was difficult. I didn't stop to figure out why, or how I could change course. I just kept making the same mistakes and going through my own small version of hell.

In 2014, my pain got too much to hold any more after my marriage fell apart. I began exploring my pain with a life coach and psychologist. This was incredibly helpful and provided me with a great starting point on my journey. Eventually, I found deeper and more wholistic approaches to opening to my pain and removing my distorted beliefs, which would prove to have more sustainable outcomes for the way I feel.

That is not meant to denigrate the work that psychologists or life coaches do. They provide important services to those people with mental health challenges and my psychologist helped me a lot. Their highly skilled assistance helped me to become more mindful and emotionally secure. I discovered some of the core limiting beliefs that were holding me back in life. Many of these had been derived from my experiences growing up in a highly conditioned environment, so I had absorbed them and, as I had a strong mind, I had mastered many of these less-than-ideal beliefs.

Once I started down my path, I also learned to express my emotions and the power of my tears, and felt myself stepping through a series of different phases over the nine years of self-exploration. It was like peeling an onion, because not only did each one invoke more tears and emotion, but they also continually led me to new profound discoveries about a topic very dear to me. Me!

I had discovered that the pain in my body was a message of love from my soul. It was not intended to harm me, but to allow me to gain higher self-awareness and to make better and more informed choices in my life.

Eventually I discovered that I did not need my initial qualified mentors to steer me to higher levels of awareness, because my feelings were a greater and constant source of wisdom and showed me what I could explore next. All I had to do was listen to them and explore what was arising from inside me.

The biggest discovery I made during these various explorations was that, for most of my adult life, I hadn't known who or what I truly was with any real confidence. I had a personality and a story like everyone else, formed from years of living. But was that story really the one I was meant to write?

I had entered a fascinating phase of life in which I began to question everything I had ever held to be true about myself. I unleashed my natural curiosity – onto myself! This proved to be hard at times, but incredibly liberating. Every time I had a new realisation and expressed any associated pain, a day or two later I felt my sense of self-esteem lift. I saw how I was integrating these new learnings into my awareness, and it felt good.

I realised I had unknowingly let other people write the script of my life story and had essentially lost the plot by acting out the story that they wrote, or that I thought they wanted me to write. This was subconsciously causing me great stress and leading me to subrogate my life, trying to succeed at things I really did not desire. It also caused me to develop a debilitating physical disease that I was truly the architect of and had to go inward to heal.

I did not understand my own beliefs and was therefore not active in choosing my own path. I took the path of least resistance, which was to follow the advice of others, rather than trust my own self. In some ways, I now see how easy a trap this was to fall into.

I did not trust my own heart and never made the effort to connect to it. I did know my heart had desires – they fleetingly appeared when I was growing up as a child, with my heart telling me to be a doctor when I left school. But I progressively dismissed my heart, hiding it under a pile of ego-based and self-enforced obligations that told me I should do this or that because the world expected it of me, and I instead chose through logic and the encouragements of others to become an accountant. I liked my work, though never truly loved it. My mind chose my career path not my all-knowing heart.

If only I had listened to my heart, I wonder where my passion may have taken me!

It took great courage to begin my journey of self-discovery in my 50s, and to ultimately step into a newer truer me. Along the way, I discovered so many incredible new aspects of me that made me happier and helped me to relax.

Initial releases of pain came with much feeling and intense outpourings of grief. I was stunned by how much pain I had stored in my subconscious mind and body, and how old much of it was.

I welcomed these new exposures, and allowed them to come forth, constantly opening to receiving the next one, because they helped me on every level – my mind, body and soul are all now in unification, not separation, and I feel far happier and excited by life.

I also remembered some beautiful energies that I intrinsically already had within me, but had been unable to see or feel, because they were covered up by the energies of pain and fear. These energies were related to higher levels of self-worth, self-trust, self-forgiveness, self-love, and self-acceptance. As you can see, they all related to myself.

At the same time, I discarded many unwanted energies I had once held, including self-doubt, a propensity to accept suffering, and an addiction to give more to others than I felt worthy of receiving.

Many of my negative self-opinions were related to my fear of being different and standing out in the crowd. I was happy to do well, but not too well, because that could alienate me from others. So, I stayed in the energies of safety and security, choosing to repeat my mistakes rather than search for the energy that could introduce me to new possibilities of success.

If only I had understood how much negativity I had held onto during my life, I wonder how I could have changed it for the better at a much earlier age.

But I never felt any real regret along the path. I was simply grateful that I was finally discovering deeper aspects of myself – better late than never I suppose!

How Did I Find More of the Real Me?

The path to the real me was one based more on love than fear. Some people have told me they admire my courage to take the steps I have taken to find the real me, but it has been the most wonderful time of my life thus far, and I did it out of love for me, no one else. I know it will lead me to many new and wonderful experiences in the future.

My journey entailed turning to find a life I loved, not one I could simply tolerate, and hopefully one day retire from. I went in search of my heart first and foremost and put down my quest to accumulate material possessions temporarily. I was now much more interested in me acquiring me and finding the love within me.

To some extent, this has been a singular journey and involved some degree of isolation at times, because I had to go inward to discover the deeper aspects of myself. It can be done within relationships, or on your own, but there are times when being alone may give you more space to focus on you.

There was, however, an element of fear in my journey. After repeated versions of failure in my life, I wanted to transform myself before I transformed my life. In hindsight, I now see that I did not want to fail again. This was a great motivator for me to focus on finding the real and wiser me.

The awakening path is one that ultimately can lead you home to your own heart. It is no one else's happening. You can share your learnings with another, but they can never own them.

Of course, this path never ends, so you will continue to evolve for the rest of your life and beyond. As you discover more of yourself along this path it is, therefore, important to realise that you always have the opportunity to find more of yourself and what you are capable of.

There have been several different phases in my awareness journey and as you have no doubt gleaned in this book so far, I have been heavily supported by metaphysical energies. Many deny its existence in their lives, but the truth is it is ever present in every experience you go through, and it is incredibly loving, whether you choose to embrace it or not. I have never experienced a purity of love in my life that can match this love, and I continue to be supported by it through my contact with the metaphysical realms.

Embracing the metaphysical aspects of ourselves is a choice we all get to make.

Even if we ignore it and we are in resistance, we can't change the fact that we are connected to the universe, and we are not separate. Embracing it can however speed up our awakening as it allows a greater flow of love to be applied to our lives. Love is the most powerful force in any transformation.

The higher the vibration of energy you deploy and the higher the purity of love you allow yourself to be, the higher the transformation that is possible for you to co-create with the universe. The universe knows when you are committed to your own transformation, and when you release the resistance that your mind naturally wants to put up to this process, you can allow your transformation to follow its intended course.

The universe loves you more than you may ever know. In fact, it has no limits.

The Normal Way We Change

Before I delve into the Natural Arc of Human Transformation, the 'Arc', let us consider how change is normally approached in society, both on an individual level and in collectives.

This is how I changed for the first 53 years of my life and why I struggled to make real progress after major disruptions in my life. I thought I had overcome issues, but the fact is they continued to weigh me down in a myriad of pain and regret. These losses continued to aggregate as I aged, because I realised I was constantly trying to do better, with the same level of consciousness and unchanged belief structures. I think this has been referred to by some as a form of insanity!

Without any heightened self-awareness, and the intelligence that allows, the process of change is usually approached from the mind.

But our minds are typically focussed on returning us from disruption back to our perception of the normality we were used to, or where we hoped to be before the disruption and associated pain arose. We want to reach the expectations that we previously set ourselves, and enjoy the circumstances we once enjoyed, and we typically want this return to normal to be as painless and fast as possible.

This process of recovery can often result in incremental improvements, but whole new paradigms are unlikely to arise unless heightened self-awareness is also attained and acted upon, because without such we do not have the full power of consciousness behind us, and thus the way we feel is unlikely to substantially change for the better.

Without such wisdom, normal approaches to change often involve the deflection of blame onto others and the propensity not to take responsibility for issues that we have had a hand in. These are all attributes of an unhealthy but normally functioning ego, which seeks to protect and promote the person it purports to serve. I use the word 'purports' because the ego can be a great hinderance in us making exponential leaps forward in our lives.

The blame game, for instance, can block us from accessing learning opportunities that might open the door to significant paradigm shifts, and improvements in our circumstances. With the blame game so securely entrenched in our society, blame can even morph into shame, and shame is an awful energy for anyone to carry through life.

This is fundamentally different to the experience that is possible through the Arc. In the Arc, we get to turn to our core operating system: the intuitive centre within us. Here, we can open to new possibilities, consider what arises, and look for exponential, not incremental, improvements by connecting to the higher awareness within us. Putting the Arc into operation requires patience and deep trust in ourselves, rather than in the normal ways change is approached in society.

In 1969, Dr Elizabeth Kubler-Ross introduced the world to what she called the five stages of grief. Her findings were inspired by deep enquiry into the subject of death, and how humans respond to such an event; but could also be applied to far less significant forms of disruption, such as a loss of status, freedom, relationships, or money. At a societal or business organisation level, disruptions such as these can be incredibly stressful for many, particularly where it leads to a deep sense of failure for those involved.

The five states of grief (or emotion) that Kubler-Ross established are commonly referred to as being:

1. Denial
2. Anger
3. Bargaining
4. Depression
5. Acceptance

These five stages are well documented in other research materials on the internet, and I suspect that readers may have had their own experiences with them, depending on how life has unfolded.

When my personal losses arose earlier in my life, I experienced all these emotions as I struggled to cope with my perceived misfortunes.

For much of my life, I reacted to disruptions in a low conscious way that I admit was largely unsophisticated. My ability to learn from the adversity was low. My resilience I thought was high. But this turned out to be a terrible combination.

The truth was I was avoiding pain, and most of the time just trying to get back to the 'devil I knew'. I hated not having control of things in my life, unaware that control and love are polar opposites. There is truly no love in control!

I wanted the problems fixed so I could return to the situation I had gotten used to, perhaps with some minor level of enhancement, but that wasn't my priority. I just wanted the pain I was experiencing to go away – to stop now. I hated the thought of being some kind of failure.

I effectively tried to pick myself up and try again, and again, without really learning from the situation at hand and self-reflecting on how I could have been different in the circumstances that prevailed.

Surely, I didn't deserve this, I thought!

I struggled to cope with any form of failure because my levels of self-forgiveness were low. High resilience with low self-forgiveness is also not a great combination. It saw me suppress and hide my pain and led me to great personal suffering, that a more aware me could have avoided.

So, I would add the following additional contextual observations to the normal way we face personal trauma through the five stages of grief, as they provide a backdrop for my more natural way to confront unexpected losses:

- Blame: where possible we try to protect and promote ourselves from blame during a personal crisis. The intensity of the blame game we play is somewhat influenced by our personal self-esteem levels, and the relative strength of our egos.

High ego people with artificially high self-esteem are more likely to 'sheet home' blame to others, and not accept their rightful contribution to a disruption or problem.

The secure person with healthy self-esteem is likely to see the situation with greater objectivity, and only accept the blame that is rightfully theirs to own. They are more in the energy of self-love.

People with unhealthy egos that lead them to low self-esteem, may take the blame that is not theirs to hold. This is fear based.

The presence of blame is not helpful in a disruptive time for it belies the opportunities for learning, that may be possible. When any issues arise that are less than ideal, particularly within a relationship, it's always important to go inward to your heart and consider how you may have contributed to a problem first before you go outward to find some other party to blame.

A mirror exists in many problematic situations between two people, such as in a marriage breakdown, and this mirror provides a great opportunity for both parties to see how their actions or beliefs may have contributed to a dysfunction.
Of course, it can take great courage to be willing to go inward and discover how you could have made a more positive contribution to any situation. The person who can do this is most likely of high integrity.

- Doing: when we find ourselves in an unwanted situation our temptation is to do what is necessary to return to normal. This can be fair in some cases, but it is also important to be with your feelings as problems unfold, for these feelings can change our energy in a situation and alter what we subsequently decide to do. Many breakdowns involve feelings and probably can't be readily fixed by just doing something to fix the problem. We must honour our feelings by giving them the opportunity to be processed and properly interpreted. Then we can act upon them. This requires us to give our feelings, including pain, space in which they can be felt and heard.

- Depression: *I have experienced my own version of depression in my life. I was extremely resilient; but, because I was out of alignment with my own true self for much of my life, I suffered significant stress. This stress did not manifest as clinical depression, but it manifested as the debilitating muscle disorder that severely impacted my life. If I had understood what I know now and have written into this book, I am sure I would have experienced much less worry in my life. As a result, I would have been much happier and healthier.*

As we age, our sense of failure can aggregate off the back of disruptions and losses that we have incurred and weigh us down. This can push us from sadness to depression because, essentially, we lose faith in life. The hopes and dreams we held so dear as a younger version of ourselves, have not been met and we can spiral into a place where we feel it's easier to just give up. But this sense of wanting to give up is just another form of control. We are not surrendering to what is, learning new ways of being and approaching our lives with the fresh perspectives that higher intelligence can make possible. We are in resistance to new possibilities.

It is time we approached pain in a more natural way to end the epidemic of depression and worry that are so rife in our society. Surrender and acceptance are great antidotes for depression, as my own story depicts.

- Grief: the five stages of grief place acceptance as the final step to recovery. However, the level of acceptance we achieve is often distorted by our minds and is not real or fully achieved. We just think it is.

In some situations, we may think that we have reached a point of acceptance that is healthy, and so we can move on with our lives. But *are* we really over the event and its consequences that impacted upon us, or did we just suppress and bury some of the pain that poured forth in the experience?

After my second divorce I felt pain for years. I thought I was free of the pain, but it lingered within me until I learned to process it fully and see the positives and purpose of the marriage breakdown I had endured. My pain did not go away until I understood and felt the gifts of awareness that had arisen from my divorce, and effectively allowed my heart and body to process my grief. This required great releases of my pain, and not just the process of thinking my way to a release. Thinking alone can never truly allow you to fully process pain as I found out.

Everything in life has pluses and minuses when we consider them objectively.

Self-Forgiveness is Critical

We are good at thinking that we have reached a point of forgiveness for ourselves or others. However, true forgiveness can't be thought; it must be felt and embodied in our whole selves.

Disruption that is not fully processed through the release of pain, will invariably lead us to accumulate unreconciled fears and negative beliefs that can hold us back as our lives unfold.

I found this in romantic relationships after my two divorces. With the benefit of hindsight, there was a part of me that lost trust in any relationship working again. This subconscious fear led me, to some extent, into a place of self-sabotage, because I felt that no long-term relationship could ever work for me again.

Opening to and addressing this destructive belief was only made possible by my subsequent journey into higher consciousness. I had to fully release the pain I was carrying, so that I could identify the limiting beliefs that were holding me back. I did not want to be alone as much as I was, but my fears led me there subconsciously until I discovered them. Essentially, my pain helped me to become free.

I eventually came to see that my heart had allowed me to venture into loving situations. It was the distorted beliefs and fears in my mind that had ruined the potential for love to flourish.

Our world is full of broken hearts, owned by people who never fully recovered from the destructive beliefs that were created by trauma. They have held on to suffering and grief arising from a situation, and no amount of reasoning or thinking has been able to set them free. Their pain has become an intrinsic part of them and is most likely still harming their wellbeing and ageing them physically as a result.

The heart-based magic inherent in the journey to higher self-awareness through the natural process I call the Arc, makes a full recovery possible, and so much more.

The normal way society has taught us to process grief is full of mind-based reactions and responses. It allows little possibilities for us to arise to higher heights from the ashes of despair. It is devoid of many realities of how life truly works and does not lend itself to expansion and the discovery of new and exciting possibilities, for it views pain and disruption through the lens of bad or evil, not opportunity.

This belies the truth of life: that disruption happens *for* us and *through* us, not *to* us. Once you truly own this statement you can't help but change the quality of your life.

The traditional perception of pain is out of sync with universal realities, and contributes to our obsession with *pain management* rather than *pain consciousness*, and blocks us from recognising the vital role pain can have in leading us home to ourselves.

The ego may tell us we have risen above the situation. But have we really? Only our feelings are able to give us this answer, and this requires us to deeply open ourselves up to their messages of love. They are our source of truth.

If there is any residual pain and limited learning, we have *not* fully transcended the issue. By applying the Arc, we both learn from and overcome fear.

If you believe you have a propensity to accept suffering and hang onto pain in your life, it is likely that the natural process to transform your life that the Arc puts forward will bring you a brighter future.

When we merely seek to recover from disruption in our lives, and not use it as a springboard to discover new heights, we deny ourselves the chance to learn more about what lies within us and make us truly happy.

Why just manage your pain and begrudge it for the rest of your life, when you can instead turn pain into power?

Bring your pain into your light for it's not here to be managed. It's here to illuminate your possibilities.

Opportunity awaits those who climb their springboard and dive into a whole new paradigm; one where you can float freely on a sea of endless support from the universe!

CHAPTER 12

The Natural Arc of Human Transformation

The Secure Bridge Between Your Future and Your Past

My personal transformation has left me with the knowing that, if any major losses or disruptions ever 'grace' my life again, they will be greeted by a much more aware and composed me, who will deal with them much faster and comprehensively, and release any associated pain very quickly. I will transcend the pain that arises, by opening to it, loving its wisdom, and going through it and beyond.

The gap between the you-that-may-be-suffering, and the you-that-will-not, can be found when you embrace the Arc of your own personal transformation. This is a completely natural process through which we can all find new possibilities. And guess what – it is free, unlike trips to mental health professionals and drugs.

You've heard of Noah's Ark and the Ark of the Covenant. The story of Noah's Ark is a representation of rebirth following a massive flood, allowing mankind and the animal kingdom to experience new beginnings. The Ark of the Covenant reputably held the tablets that gave humanity the 10 commandments spoken of by Moses. Both Arks gave humanity fresh hope and direction.

The Arc I have built may be spelt slightly differently, but it gives you, the reader, a new way to find your truth, your light and in turn new possibilities that you can create.

It looks like this:

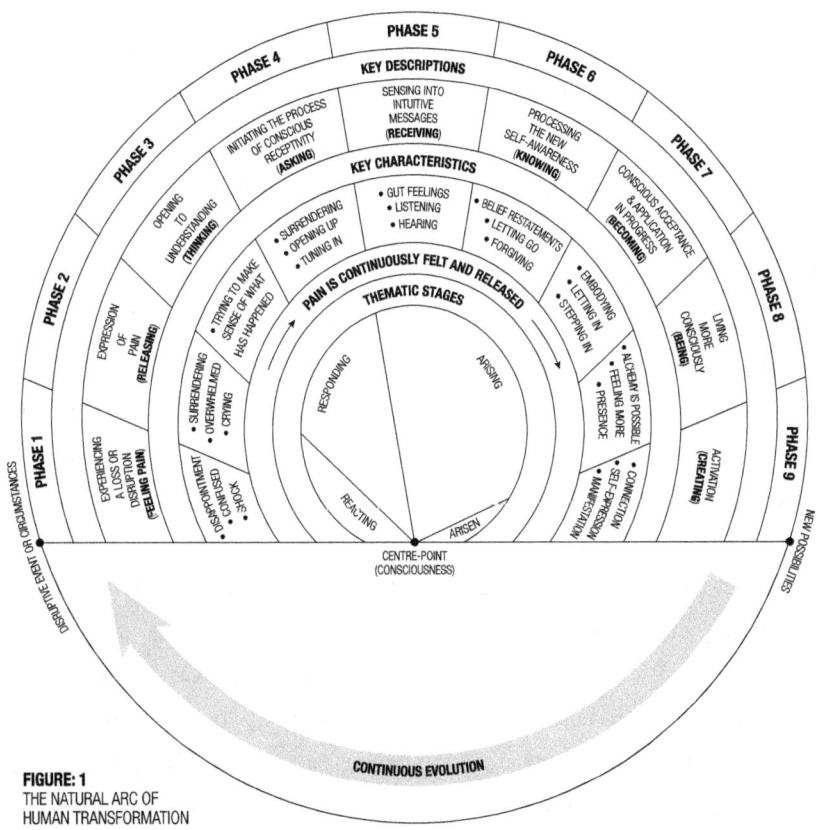

FIGURE: 1
THE NATURAL ARC OF
HUMAN TRANSFORMATION

The key phases of this natural process can permanently change your very being. Once you start regularly applying them, waves of changes will result in a profound transformation of your self-esteem.

The Arc operates primarily through pure consciousness, with support from your IQ and body. It can be applied to all sources of confusion or pain, big or small. Once it is applied consistently and becomes a fundamental part of the way you remove pain and upgrade your conditioned belief structures, it will raise the vibration of your very being, such that you will open the door for your true self to become the architect of your entire life. And in the process, you will build a temple that can stand strong until you pass to your next adventure!

This is a progressive happening and at some stage the more advanced participants will burst forth, becoming their wholistic, creative self, capable of manifesting the life they dream about. This is the magic of Phase 9, and the place where great spiritual masters have arrived.

You can join them!

Your true self can burst forth when you have done the 'work' to bring your vibration in alignment with your loving soul. It will respond to your commitment to becoming the real you and respond accordingly, because it is the essence of you. However, this will only occur when the universe knows you are ready for such an event, not when you hope or think you are.

The number nine in spirituality represents the end of a cycle. The last phase of the Arc in Phase 9 is a powerful possibility that awaits you. Sitting in the light in this phase is your radiant self, ready to manifest at will what your heart desires. Here you become advanced normality – no better than anyone else, just a person who is truly in their own light and being what God intended.

In this magical place you become the creator you were born to be – the alchemist, who is fully transformed and able to be more than just a conscious person. In this place, you become a vessel for the reimagining of your own life for your soul and will stand as a representation for others of what is possible when you surrender to your truth and love. The light will work through you. You will be vibrant because you will BE the vibration of universal love, fully aware of your light and able to Earth it into your life.

This is your holy grail, and your cup will overflow with love and the access to higher intelligences that will grace your presence.

Practical Aspects of the Arc

Like anything in life, you will master the Arc the more you apply it and move deeper into it. Businesses speak of continuous improvement in how they operate. They undertake this activity as a matter of course. This can also apply to you when you understand the natural way you can live and expand your way through life.

As you continue to apply the Arc, you will get deeper and deeper into knowing its full potential. As you move through its phases your personal vibration and inherent self-awareness will rise, enabling you to reap greater benefits and apply it more fully. You will become more advanced, particularly in hearing, interpreting, and applying the wisdom of your own heart. This is likely to change your life circumstances for the better, even before you get to more advanced phases.

There are no rules as to the speed at which you can or will move through the Arc and progressively apply it. If you have limited conditioning or karma, you may move to advanced phases easily or, in fact, already be there. You may be beyond it, like some advanced souls that have walked this planet.

Alternatively, the latter stages of the Arc may initially be out of your reach. For example, the ability to manifest through the soul is quite advanced. It took me nearly nine years to enter Phase 9!

Let's consider another example. As you enter Phase 5 of the Arc and learn to receive messages from your soul you will gradually grow in confidence as to how your heart communicates with you. Do you hear words, or intuitive feelings, or experience both?

From my experience, the speed at which you receive these messages will also lift from days then to hours, and eventually to minutes. And the way you receive messages can vary and evolve. Mine went from feelings to whispers, to profound messages I now hear constantly in my head.

You will start to learn how the universe brings forth synchronicity for you to step into, and you will become more accustomed to changing your belief structures to facilitate whatever change you need.

A phase like Phase 6 (i.e. Knowing) could take you months or years to master. Everyone's natural aptitude will vary. I took years to master Phase 6 because my ability to let go and truly trust my true self was blocked by my strong yet stubborn mind. But a less conditioned person may be more adept in this space.

If you can reach Phase 6 in the initial periods of applying the Arc, and at least hear or feel and interpret snippets of truth from your heart, you will start to reap benefits, even if you have not yet mastered other aspects of this phase. But with perseverance you will enter more advanced stages. The more effective you are at getting your ego out of the way of the truth as it arises, the faster you will progress.

The role your mind plays as you apply the Arc will shift gradually as it becomes more accustomed to its role as the assistant and interpreter, rather than the owner of your inner wisdom. You don't want to know what your mind already knows. That just places you in a limiting loop. You are searching to apply the previously unheard wisdom of your soul. This takes a bit of getting used to!

You will grow as you start to know yourself. The Arc evolves with you as you evolve, allowing you to build a bridge from the old you to the emerging you.

Applying the Arc to your life will most likely challenge you significantly. It requires a high level of commitment, and the integrity to be able to face your truths. It leads you to your truth, but requires truth to be the backbone of this application by you. It is a conscious way of living based on the accessing of higher consciousness that your soul already has. That's why I call it a journey of remembrance.

To apply it fully, will literally need you to face the demons you once called truth, but as they step out of the shadows you will come to see them as the illusions they truly are – figments of your imagination and your karmic past. They may be honest thoughts, but as we discussed earlier honesty can have stark limits when compared to truth.

Now, let's consider each phase of the Arc in detail:

Phase 1 – Experiencing a Loss or Disruption (Feeling Pain)

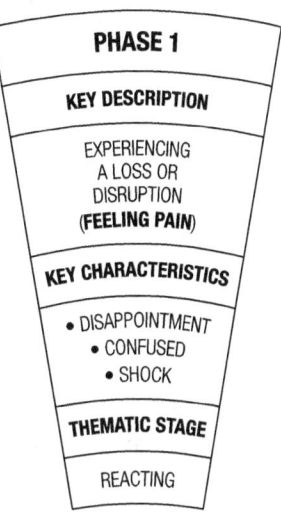

Many disruptions in our lives can lead to us seeing them as some form of loss. We have not got we hoped for or expected, and we experience pain. This can send us into turmoil and create unwanted emotions within our senses, leading us to energies of shock, disappointment, despair, revenge, blame, and so on.

Most people only see the bad in these types of events, and seek to return to their old 'normal' as soon as possible. The ego does not like being challenged in this way because there is often a perceived loss of status, image, or wellbeing. They believe the loss has happened *to* them and they enter the limiting five stages of grief.

My book *Where Your Happiness Hides* gives a deeper account of this process for interested readers. Essentially, as we try and prove that we are lovable in life, every failure we encounter reinforces our belief that we are not able to be loved, despite this being truly impossible. Success gives us short term relief from our dilemma, but our illusions can lead us ever closer to the pain of the belief that we are not enough. Eventually, we can crack and feel like giving up. This can be the root of depression and misery.

However, the conscious person can take a very different route through the circumstances to one of expansion and new levels of self-awareness. They know that the disruption has happened *for* and *through* them, and circumstances will present new beginnings for them to enjoy – if they approach them in a conscious and curious way. They accept that the human being who they are, finds the altered circumstances uncomfortable, and perhaps shocking. They can and most likely will feel disappointment and pain. This is both normal and healthy. To do otherwise can be abnormal. Emotions are there for our benefit and the associated pain is our indicator that we need something to change.

But all has purpose in life, including bad experiences; so, the conscious person understands that the problems they face are a gift of sorts. Our souls orchestrate events such as these to provide us with opportunities to expand and grow. The reality is, we always get what we need in life so we can return to a place of higher awareness and self-esteem. From this place we can get what we want in a more sustainable way.

The first step in the Arc is therefore to face the disruption that has taken place and not hide from it. Suppressing it will not help. It will just delay your eventual freedom from the situation and the benefits that lie within your conscious reaction.

Phase 1 is primarily a mental stage with anguish also being felt in the body because of the disappointments and torment.

In Phase 1, you are merely reacting to what has taken place or is likely to occur.

Phase 2 – Initial Release of Pain and Emotions (Expressing)

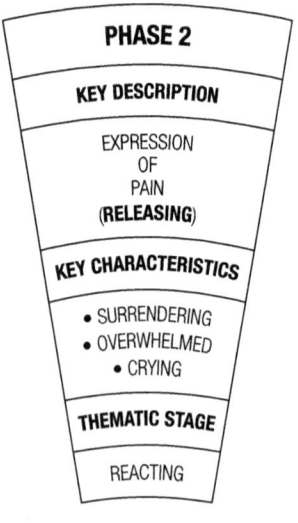

The healthy reaction to any pain your body experiences, is to express it as soon as possible. If it is left in your body, it can, and most likely will, damage your body and energy fields. The longer it stays there, the more this damage is likely to be.

You need to release your pain without judgement of yourself or anyone else, for it does not serve you to go outward and project your pain at others or inflict it upon yourself, until you have fully reconciled it and embodied its intended learnings. You are unlikely to have reached that point in Phase 2 of the Arc.

I have found great relief in allowing my pain to express itself in private once it arises, or with a close loved one who cares. I usually find a private space and let my pain out. I also allow it to talk to me, for the outbursts of the mind to that painful event, or realisation, always give me a clear picture of how my ego is reacting to the matters arising in my life or my periphery. I simply observe the outburst of my mind. This nearly always steers me towards whatever limiting beliefs that I need to address.

Playing the witness to what is expressed is very informative and allows you to see your pain and emotions as temporary but important 'visitors' from which you can learn. Outward expression of your pain is very helpful as it allows you to observe your ego's often distorted messages. This practice tends to eliminate the filters that you may otherwise impose upon the conditioned outpourings. When the ego is expressing itself, it will normally speak in the first person with lots of I's and me's.

In doing so, it is separating itself from those who you think may have harmed you unfairly, for the ego always sees itself as the limited separate self in this world, and therefore in a vulnerable place.

Pain and emotions are just energies, and the human body is not meant to hold these energies for extended periods. Energies are meant to move. They are not meant to be fixed. And every human being has the means to allow it to pass through them. In this way, emotions are energies requiring motion. They should not be feared but embraced as helpful.

The more we allow our emotions to overwhelm us in Phase 2, the greater the levels of relief we will eventually experience. The natural processes at our disposal, like crying and screaming, allow us to feel freer to then approach our problems in a calmer way.

The releasing of energies is often not limited to one single event. Depending on the severity of the disruption, like the death of a loved one or a marital breakdown, it may need to be released on multiple occasions.

My experience was that the pain of an event returned on multiple occasions as my self-awareness levels arose from within me. As my ability to surrender to the pain grew, so did the strength of the release that I felt.

One release will rarely resolve the energetic impacts of a major happening. The energy will come forth to be dealt with when you are ready and able to deal with it. Your inner sense knows when this is the case.

If pain and suffering is not released, and the subconscious mind holds associated fears and beliefs of betrayal, this pain and suffering can linger for a lifetime. It can hold a negative belief until the day you die. As I said above, time will not heal your subconscious mind; only experiences and your attention can do that. The associated energies must be dealt with.

Phase 2 is focussed on the mind and its impact on your feelings. Your mind will create the pain inside you because it is not comfortable with the situation you, or others you care for, have been placed into. Contrary to normal vernacular expressions and our understandings, the soul or heart does NOT break. Only our minds and the expectations they have created shatter in our moments of distress.

Phase 2 is about reacting to your situation.

Phase 3 – Opening to Understanding (Thinking)

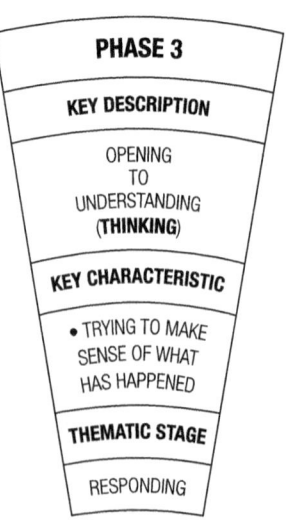

Understanding is always a mental process. When you have been impacted by a disruption or unfortunate event you will feel the shock and pain of the circumstances and try to make sense of what has taken place.

Your mind will explore the circumstances and may attempt to look for ways to take you through the five stages of grief, as discussed above. While the mind tries, however, the soul never needs to, for it has the infinite power of love and its associated wisdom within it.

But if you go down the normal path of grief, and allow your mind to torture you along the way, your mind can turn wants into non-negotiable needs, and put you into a difficult loop of pain.

The more conscious you become the more you can deflect your mind away from that unfortunate process, because the truth is that this process is unnecessary. It may be the normal way we act, but it will not serve you to move forward in a constructive way. Your mind is prone to put you into a spiral or loop of misery in which it constantly seeks relief, and relitigates the situation at hand. Hence depression descends upon your mind and can wreak havoc on your body.

When you grasp the concept that everything happens for a reason, and it is always for your benefit, as hard as this may be to get your mind around, the processing of pain takes a very different perspective and Phase 3 becomes quite short. It can liberate you to move through the problem at hand with a much more balanced perspective.

When we face an issue front on and learn our lessons, the likelihood of them recurring is also greatly diminished for we are wiser, and our energy will no longer attract those circumstances into our lives.

This has now given me great encouragement to face my issues as soon as I can, every time they arise.

Phase 3, when undertaken by a conscious person, involves their minds being the witness of the problem at hand and handing it over to their soul or intuition to provide the insights that are truly needed to move them through the problem. Consider this process to be like triage in a hospital.

The soul can never suffer, what we call, mental health problems – it simply cannot. It is way above the mind in its conscious awareness. Our problems always reside in the egoic mind!

When I experience an emotional situation these days, I do not let my mind linger or ponder the problem for very long. My mind, at my direction, relinquishes its role in solving the issue, and plays a support role in relaying the situation to my heart and interpreting the response. I may release pain and emotions, but I consider this to be important for my health and my desire to overcome the pain. This effectively leads me quickly into Phase 4 of the Arc – with a degree of anticipation, because I love improving my self-awareness levels!

We can try and hide from a painful situation by divorcing ourselves as much as possible from any blame. However, the mere fact that we are feeling pain, must mean that we are involved and have most likely contributed to the situation. Our role in the issue at hand must be owned and dealt with, or it will consume and own us.

Taking responsibility for our pain is a core step in our recovery process and the respective phases of the Arc.

After my second marriage ended, I was able to consider and tune into the beliefs and behaviours I had held that probably contributed to the divorce. I didn't just go to blame, I went deeply inward. If anything, I took far too much responsibility for the marriage ending, but at least I learned that about myself as well.

Phase 3 in a consciously growing person is therefore brief. It effectively results in the matter being considered and handed over to our intuitive hearts to find out what is truly at play.

Phase 3 is undertaken in the mind, but we need to remind our minds that it is only the interpreter and coordinator of our journey to higher awareness, not the source of wisdom that will solve our dilemma.

Phase 3 is an initial step out of reacting to our pain and onto the path of responding.

Phase 4 – Initiating the Process of Conscious Receptivity (Asking)

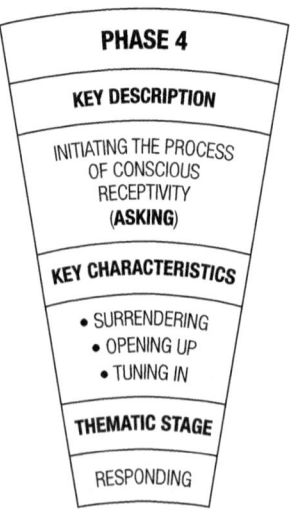

Consciousness is more than thinking. It involves the interplay of our hearts, minds, and bodies. Our minds play an important role, as discussed above, as the witness and interpreter, but unhealthy egos do not. They are destructive of the process of expansion.

So, what is conscious receptivity?

Some people might align this with meditation or tuning in to the wisdom of the soul. At any stage of our lives, our souls know what we need to expand to our next level of conscious awareness. They know what life lessons we need, and are involved in orchestrating our circumstances, so that we get the chance to progress.

You can consider yourself to be like a musical instrument that is capable of all kinds of tunes and melodies. The songs we play will be determined by who or what plays us – the ego or the soul. The soul knows what vibrations we are truly capable of bringing to this world, and the musical scores we can then create. It is intent on creating harmony within us and then between us and the outside world we inhabit.

The quieting of the mind is important to allowing the soul to express itself. This is why many people use meditation to find peace in difficult situations. This practice is important in the early stages of applying the Arc.

As I have progressed in my consciousness journey, I have felt less and less compelled to go into deep meditation to tune into my inner knowing, because my biased ego has been substantially tamed. I sit is silence and ask my soul for its wisdom with respect to a problem and I await the answer with patience. My mind knows its place and has become adept as the servant of my soul. In a way, I now meditate every minute of the day while I proceed through my physical life.

When I first started this process, the responses from my soul were slow to be sensed. Sometimes they took a day or two to be received with clarity. Sometimes my mind would attempt to interject, believing that it had all the answers and distort the process. I have a strong enquiring mind, which can be a double-edged sword in such situations.

These days, I receive the answers in minutes, even seconds. At the start of using the Arc, this could take hours and even days; so a reader should not be discouraged if they don't get fast insights.

Tuning in or going inward to self-reflect on a dilemma is a core and natural skill that we all possess. It's just a matter of remembering an incredible ability that we all possess. And like anything of value in life, it takes practice to improve our ability to do it. Essentially, we become what we practice.

Conscious receptivity is a skill you can develop, if you make time to do so. It's part of our natural abilities. You are the only person who can hear the answers from your own heart. No one else can. Others may have a view, but unless they are an incredibly evolved being of high consciousness this is not possible.

The kind of questions I often ask my heart when in Phase 4 include:

- *How do I find peace in this situation?*
- *Show me what I need to see, do, and understand in this experience.*
- *What are you wanting me to learn or change?*
- *What limiting beliefs have led me to this uncomfortable place, and which ones do I need to change or confront to create improved circumstances in my life?*
- *What actions do I need to take to avoid suffering in this situation?*
- *What attachments or validations of the mind have led me to this situation?*

Phase 4 is akin to your mind tuning into a radio station and listening to the programme that's being transmitted. Your soul is the station and can send you the news you are longing to hear.

The best energies to adopt in Phase 4 relate to that of surrender and relaxation. When we let go, relax, feel and ask our hearts for guidance we are far more likely to hear the responses with clarity.

When we ask for help, we relinquish our ego centric belief that our minds know it all. In this place, control is replaced by an open heart and a receptive mind.

Phase 4 is another form of response to our problems. Once we hear the wisdom in later phases, our energy of response can give way to the phenomena I call *arising*.

Phase 5 – Sensing into Intuitive Messages (Receiving)

Phase 5 of the Arc is a receiving phase. We have asked our consciousness or soul in Phase 3 for advice, then in Phase 4 we have trusted the process and listened, now in Phase 5 we get ready to receive it and facilitate an energy of knowing.

From my experience, the answer or answers always come in Phase 5.

It's about patiently waiting and opening for the response and having the integrity to accept the truth of your heart. It may be uncomfortable for you to hear what it wants to tell you and, therefore, your ego may encourage you to reject the advice that is on offer.

PHASE 5
KEY DESCRIPTION
SENSING INTO INTUITIVE MESSAGES (RECEIVING)
KEY CHARACTERISTICS
• GUT FEELINGS • LISTENING • HEARING
THEMATIC STAGE
ARISING

The knowing I speak of comes from feeling into the new awareness that comes through you, for you. From my experience, it is always the truth, and it is presented to you out of pure love. Your body will react with feeling, normally in the pit of your stomach, and it will confirm what you have heard, for it is from the seat of consciousness inside you. This is often referred to as a gut feeling.

You may receive messages from your soul as such feelings, or in the form of words that you register in your brain. Some may receive both. We are all different.

You will know the difference between wisdom from your heart and the information coming from your ego. The soul does not repeat itself unless you ask again. It is direct and definite, and the response may feel uncompassionate, because it is relaying truth to your interpreting mind. It can be almost blunt, but it is always clear. The truth may hurt, but it is truly the only place from which to start a transformation.

A message from the mind is different. As I previously touched on, it may repeat itself, argue with itself and relitigate what it thinks is true. There can be confusion and a defensive tone. It gives you understanding. and its own form of honesty – but honesty is often very different to truth, unless they are derived from the same source.

We then need to go into the process of considering the wisdom. This means searching objectively inside of us to find what course of action we should ideally undertake. A knowing will arise if you are in integrity and authenticity when considering the response.

Phase 5 is a soul-based activity, with your mind assisting with the interpretation and knowing. The open heart has the knowing, and it relays it to the open mind.

Phase 5 is your first foray into the energy of arising. Arising is different to rising. You will feel the arising coming up from within you as your truth starts to come forth and take you to higher consciousness. Rising is an ego-based concept. It is designed to raise your status or self-image.

Phase 6 – Processing the New Self-Awareness (Knowing)

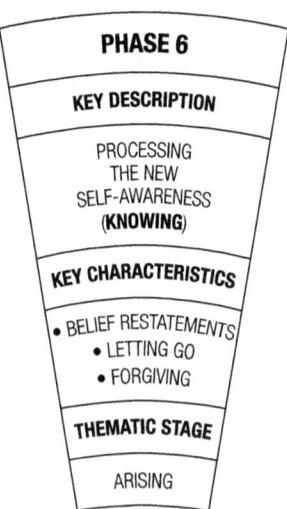

In Phase 6, we have received the truth of a situation from our consciousness by connecting to our inner-senses, or purity. And this will have stimulated a knowing in us about what needs to change in our beliefs and energies. They are closely related.

But just knowing the truth of a

situation and having a plan to address it, is not enough to create the change that is required. There are steps ahead to free yourself of the old attachments, energies and beliefs that may have been holding you back.

I spoke of the unlearning process that is so critical in attaining higher awareness. It comes into play at this stage. Once you have identified the beliefs that need to change, you must let them go. By letting go you allow space for new energies and beliefs to arise within you, and to essentially become a part of you.

In my book *Where Your Happiness Hides*, I provided a deeper understanding of the way the universe interacts with our beliefs to bring us the opportunity to attain higher awareness. Essentially, the universe through the unlimited power of your soul, knows exactly what limiting beliefs you hold in any moment. It can do this because the soul is your eternal being.

When you are deemed to be ready to face and change a limiting belief, your soul will allow circumstances to arrange themselves around you, to bring forth the awareness you need to understand. It acts as a mirror and gives you what you need, to enable you to question and clear the limiting beliefs you hold. This can feel harsh at times, depending on the events and feelings that arise, but it is a core reason why you are here on this Earth now, and having the experiences that you are involved with – to help you to expand and move closer to being your true loving self.

By embracing the circumstances that arise and witnessing the impact of your beliefs, you can choose to transcend them and advance the circumstances of your life, and how you feel about them. The universe always gives you what you need in this process, by manifesting your fears into reality. Once you overcome your energies of need, you can manifest what you want.

Normally when an experience involves more than one person, all involved receive the experiences and feelings that they need to help them grow. But others involved in an experience you are having may not be aware of this gift. That doesn't matter, for you have the power to focus on your own awareness. Remember you are living your life, not theirs.

Letting go of your old 'baggage' can be difficult, particularly if your ego is in resistance. This is very normal. Letting go of the personality your mind has spent years creating and trying to protect and promote is no small task – although it can be, once you master the Arc. You need to essentially get out of the way of the truth that is wanting to infiltrate you to stimulate the expansion that you need.

Forgiveness of self and others is a vital part of this process. At different stages you will realise that the conditioned beliefs that you held, caused you much damage in your life or had the potential to.

In my awakening process, I found thousands of conditioned beliefs I needed to discard, although I did use some experts to help me find them, by helping me to unwind my experiences and do what I called sparking my dark.

My experiences in Phase 6 were instrumental in my formulation of my book on core limiting human belief structures, **Where Your Happiness Hides.**

Your temptation, once you see yourself more clearly and recognise your role in your own demise, will be to 'beat yourself up' or resent others for their involvement. You may come to see, like I did, that some of your beliefs were unfounded and destructive. They may also have arisen from the views or actions of others who influenced your life. Some may have been destructive experiences that you could not avoid. This may include your parents, relatives, teachers, or even the media you were drawn to or forced to observe as you grew up.

Forgiveness of yourself and others for what has happened, as I said above, is a critical part of your expansion. When you witness the truth, you should ideally not let it inflate or deflate your perceptions of the worthiness of yourself or others. But this is easier said than done because your mind can be a formidable foe.

Experiences that have taken place can gift you the gift of self-awareness if you are vigilant to that possibility. Perhaps that self-awareness has arrived many months or years later than the event itself; however, time is not as critical as the mere fact that you have seen the truth. You will never see what you are meant to witness until you are ready to receive it. That is how the journey to higher consciousness works.

If you do not forgive yourself or others for your respective roles in an experience, you are in denial of one of the key tenants of the journey to consciousness – that all that arises happens for you and through you. Nothing is a random experience or can be attributed to luck.

Indeed, we often see misfortune as a bad thing, or a punishment, coming from bad luck or the forces of evil. This is never the case. You can either learn from misfortune and move towards your intended path, or take your chances in the shaky arms of regret.

The day I stopped believing that the mishaps in my life were just unlucky, was the day I moved towards my truth. I had all the wrong experiences and relationships that I needed to show me my damaging beliefs and attachments! As I tuned in to the truth through the Arc, I took more and more positive steps forward, and experienced less and less bitterness.

Only your ego will ever want or seek pity and revenge. Your loving heart will not.

Your heart will revel in any new beliefs you can now adopt and the attachments you can release, for it has arranged the experiences to assist you in concert with other souls. Sometimes you simply must pay for learnings in life. Ideally you are able to receive them when you are open to dealing with them constructively.

I did, without doubt, during my two divorces. I took deep learnings from both and I'm grateful for that now, even though both events caused me great pain, suffering and material losses at the time that they took place.

Forgiveness is always for the person giving the forgiveness, not the one it is directed at. Essentially that other party may not care what you think or feel. If your own mind was in a place of delusion because of an experience, you must forgive it and yourself. It was only responding to the environment it was placed into, using the memories it possesses. It did its best!

Often the more enquiring minds are the ones most impacted in an unfortunate set of circumstances, because they soak up the energies that are present more readily. Less aware people can be less sensitive in difficult circumstances and may be less effected by conditioned beliefs that are imposed upon them. Or perhaps they do not have a desire to evolve further and therefore to delve into their conscious and unconscious beliefs.

Empathic personalities may also be more impacted by situations that arise, for example in the case of conflicts, because their compassion for others is so high. Reactions are therefore variable, depending on our beliefs and associated energies.

The important part of Phase 6 is that you recognise your need to change a belief, relationship or attachment, and you commit to doing so. There may be more pain in the release that takes place as old energies pass through you. It is important to allow this further releasing to take place so that old redundant beliefs can exit your mind, field and ultimately your body's cellular structure in divine timing. Remember your mind cannot do this alone.

Releasing a belief by going inward, for instance in meditation, can assist greatly with the process of embodiment, but it must be felt not just thought. The impact of a revised belief has limited impact until you embody it, in other words you own it and start to change the way you behave as a result.

Phase 6 takes place in the soul, mind, and body. Embodiment is an important stage of the Arc because new levels of awareness are beginning to be understood, known, and felt in all levels of our being at once.

We now have the self-awareness, and we are owning it, however it is still possible that we will continue to walk our path in line with our old patterns of behaviour. This is conquered in later phases.

Phase 6 is an important part of our arising.

Phase 7 – Conscious Acceptance and Application (Becoming)

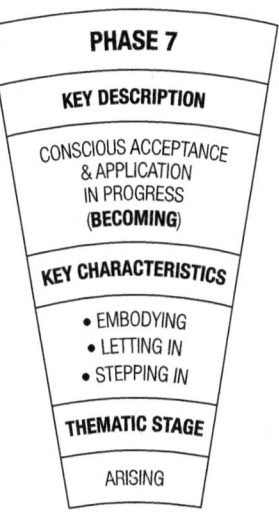

We will always be tested by the universe, through our own souls, to ensure that we become what we are now ready to become. The passage to higher consciousness must not just be understood and known, it must be applied before it is fully integrated. We must *become* pure of heart in the physical before we are able to merge with our metaphysical divinity.

In this phase, your heart, mind, and body are in sync, or integrated with each other. In other words, what you know, understand, feel and do are all in alignment. The body feels, the mind thinks, and the heart knows. Together, they then act. Our heart-based beliefs drive our feelings, which drive our thoughts, which initiate our actions. This is the natural path to creation. There are no questions within you because you just are what you are. You know what you stand for, and you stand for it.

The common bond between all these energies is always love. When you are in alignment with the heart and your ego is dissolving, you move closer to being, or vibrating in and as the energy of love. The universe supports this form of co-creation in perpetuity.

As your awareness grows, you still stand the risk of reintroducing an old belief or levels of awareness until you have stepped into circumstances and applied your new awareness in a practical way.

Synchronicity will always arise to test you in this, because you are in the arms of infinite intelligence, a power that is always present and supporting you through your journey.

How this works is way beyond the comprehension of any human mind!

But in a place of authenticity, you will be supported by the force of your soul. There is an advanced process available to all of us to assist in the processing of energetic releases. This is called transcendence and is facilitated by the soul.

Transcendence is a natural but advanced process, and is experienced in different ways by different people. It means to go through and beyond something, like pain. Trans as a prefix is associated with words that relate to going across or traversing something, like the word transfer. 'Cend' is a prefix aligned with words associated with rising above, like to ascend.

I discovered transcendence after about eight years of awakening, but this was made possible by my years of evolution and deep self-reflection. I discuss my practical experiences with transcendence later in this book.

Once you have applied your new wisdom, and can step into being the new, wiser you, you can also begin to let in what is truly intended, for there is space for it to flourish in the absence of the old energies.

The more you become accustomed to applying the Arc to your life, the more you will recognise tests as they arise through synchronicity. If you don't fully apply what you now know, new tests will confront you until you prove to your higher or true self that you've mastered your new energies and intentions.

Phase 7 is a fascinating phase and involves all aspects of you (i.e. mind, body, and spirit) interacting with circumstances that arise for you and through you. If you are like me, you will probably laugh when new tests arise, because you can sense what you are being tested to apply. In this energy you are becoming more in sync with the universe.

The true-you will begin to arise as you apply your new levels of awareness to real life and actual experiences. You are a spirit living a physical life until the day you die. Both aspects of your truth must be in alignment in duality before your full consciousness can burst forth and manifest into 3D reality.

Phase 7 is an important part of the arising.

Phase 8 – Living More Consciously (Being)

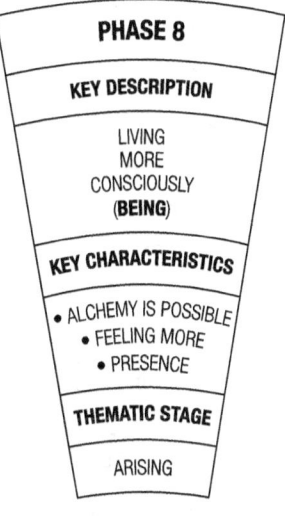

The journey through the Arc is one of going inward, then applying your new awareness outwardly. You learn and unlearn about yourself and get closer and closer to your truth. This is the natural process of personal transformation, applying aspects of yourself in the way God (or your soul), intended. Heart, mind, and body all being allowed to engage together in the capacity they naturally fulfil; not in our normal operating model with the mind shutting down your feelings and emotions, and only periodically letting you heart and bodily feelings have a say.

In a sense, you are the experiment being progressively worked on to transform you to the real you. You have been on a journey of purification. But along the way you will need to come out of your own inner laboratory to allow the new and truer you to conduct human trials with the rest of the world. You move from being through personal transformation to interacting with others in the population.

In my book *Where Your Happiness Hides*, I spoke of the natural state of being that is conducive to real happiness. I called this the Code of Happiness. When you become the true unique you and participate in harmony with the world around you, you are in your natural place to experience bliss.

There is limited benefit to you, or the world, if you become enlightened and remain in isolation. You need to be present with society and give others the benefit of your light that is gradually shining brighter for all to see. Presence is the key state of heightened awareness. It is your truth. You are pure presence. This is where love lives and where you move to being overwhelmed by the vibration of it.

As you dissolve your limiting beliefs, attachments, and fears, you will discover significant shifts in the way you feel, and the way you engage in your own life and with broader society. You initially find you become more present within yourself, and then more present with the broader population around you.

This starts to aggregate over time, and every transformative experience adds to the last to gradually lift you up. As you become more and more in the energy of your true self, you become more present with your own possibilities. You can enter a place of evolving purity in which you will begin to love life more and more. How could you not? You have love, you are love, and eventually it overwhelms you.

Other people will notice your new way of living and will be curious as to how you have become different.

Once you start to apply the Arc to the matters that worry you, you will start to employ its principles daily to all events and realisations that result in feelings within you – not just major disruptions. You will begin to see your world through the lens of truth and not illusion. You can also apply it to learn from positive situations, rather than just taking them for granted. Your life will change for the better in this phase.

I certainly started by applying it to the major issues I had encountered in my life, but I had 53 years plus of catching up to do. Now I apply it to every feeling that arises in my body. It has become automatic. In this way, my evolution has become a constant process of inner enquiry followed by outward expression. I release pain and celebrate my every lift. Not a day goes by when I don't have a new revelation about my true self or the illusions to which I still cling. I find it invigorating. You might say I have become a self-awareness junkie!

All the works of the spiritual masters that I have studied, teach that your inner reality aways becomes your outer reality. Therefore, if you want to improve the life you are experiencing on the outside, the best place to start is by changing the inner experience of yourself – your inner self-awareness, in other words.

I disagree with those so-called experts who believe that you can simply think more positively, and your life will automatically improve. It helps to some degree, because it supports a more positive vibration; but it is more of a support act to finding your inner truth through bringing your impurities to the light for cleansing.

The same goes for hypnosis. Tricking the mind without the benefit of true learning may have a placebo effect, but it is fundamentally flawed in my view because it does not involve the source of true wisdom: the soul. It's a temporary illusion and just another form of conditioning, devoid of truth.

Mind-based treatments will not work consistently, unless you have fundamentally addressed the beliefs that drive your feelings, thoughts, and actions, and feel deeply into your responses to life. Beliefs are the cornerstone of awareness and drive so much of our very being. That is why I wrote *Where Your Happiness Hides*, about human belief structures. Their power to influence our individual lives and the world we live in is vastly underrated. Rules and thoughts will never have their full force unless they are backed by beliefs.

Your thinking will likely crumble under pressure, when your limited belief structures are tested significantly, and you are not clear on what you stand for. It is often said that people will 'turn to type' or 'show their true colours' when they are put under pressure. This is because their beliefs and thoughts are not aligned in an integrated way. As a result, when fear kicks in, they are driven by their beliefs, which are normally conditioned in some less-than-ideal way. So, they abandon the values and principles that they profess to live by or plastered upon the wall, as they were just thoughts without the backing of embodied beliefs.

Once you become more self-aware, after using the Arc to evolve, you will be able to create more in your life. The experience of yourself will lift, and you will have greater clarity about what you want. Why? Because your heart is the centre of love and desire. It knows what you love and who you love. It knows what is of interest and value to you because it is free of conditioning. That's why feeling your way through life and not just thinking is so critical.

This will allow you to start crafting the life you truly want, for you will know in your heart what that is because you will be able to hear the whispers of your heart so much more clearly. More and more you will begin to exist in the energy of love.

Phase 8 is the culmination of the process of arising.

Phase 9 – Activation (Creating)

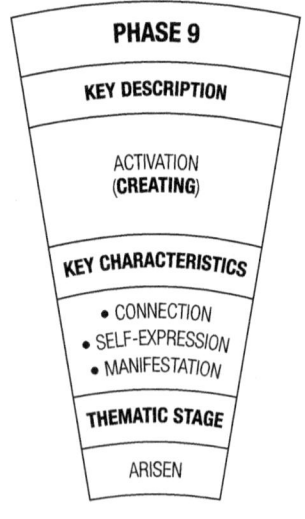

Activation is the final phase of the Arc. In this phase, you go beyond being conscious and are it-always. You are now the consciousness you originally sought. There is no separation in your mind, body, or soul to pure love, for your vibration has overwhelmed you. You are one with pure presence.

This process is essentially bestowed upon you by God. You can only invite this experience by attaining the consciousness to bring your dense energies and beliefs to the light for purification.

Human beings are natural creators, for we are creation living a human life. There are no exceptions. No one is left out of this reality.

We all have the potential to be this, for in our souls we already are. We just do not *think* we are. This wisdom has been lost through the centuries by most through countless reincarnations in which we have been exposed to suffering. We have lost the knowing of our full potentialities. Our truth has been eroded and covered up by karmic energies and pain.

Each time you remove energies getting in the way of your truth, you move closer and closer to your true self. The pace at which this takes place is one of co-creation. Your soul gives you constant opportunities to expand. You can choose how responsive you are to these opportunities. You can choose to live your life in love, or to be love and let it live you. This is our natural state.

The universe is comprised of universal love. We are that at our core. There is no separation, we just think there is.

Manifestation from your heart becomes increasingly possible when you evolve this far into the Arc. You reach the point where you are living as the creator, particularly once you have had the full incursion with your light.

You can look past your life's circumstances and allow the energy of love to embrace you. In this place, love becomes a constant source of enthusiasm and excitement for you. This powerful energetic resource is always available within you when you need it and is a powerful foundation from which to manifest.

Until you can hear or feel your heart, you will most likely be manifesting with the ideals of your mind, which can be far less potent and less supported by the universal forces of creation. Structures and interactions created from the place of ego will always be temporary in nature, for the forces of duality will dismantle them in time.

Your true self is the vibration of universal love. Therefore, what it wants to bring forth will always be in alignment with this vibration. Combining this vibration with the energy of human commitment or intention can result in wonderful creations for you.

Moving into the vibration of love is the natural foundation for an activating individual in Phase 9, to merge their light being (that is their true or eternal self) with their temporary and physical human being. This means that mind, body and spirit come into a better state of balance as the metaphysical and physical aspects establish an enhanced awareness of each other. The light being is able to fully fill the human body and energy field, and be in sync with the mind, for the individual has become highly purified, through the gradual dissolving of their ego into their wholeness.

New possibilities can arise from this new paradigm. In this place, an individual is able to become an ordinary, extraordinary person. They operate from the eternal and extraordinary wisdom of their soul, while being in their mortal and normal human form. They are likely to become more physically radiant and emotionally happy. This is an advanced way of living.

In Phase 9, an individual moves away from the inherent fear of failure, which is typical in lower states of consciousness, and enters a more inspired way of being, fully-filled with a revitalised sense of adventure for life. A preoccupation with security and safety is replaced by a desire to live with less fear and more joy.

Phase 9 is therefore all about more. As you know more and become more of your true self, you will create more. This more is created from your heart, mind and body being in a natural connection and rhythm. The more you create will be determined by your heart as you redefine what more means to you. Only you know what your heart desires. No one else but you can access this knowing and feel into what will inspire and fulfil you.

The Arc will bridge the gap between your current life and a life you almost certainly cannot even imagine - yet. Your true self knows what you are capable of and what your unique gifts to this world are. It will show you this if you use the Arc to clear the 'pipe' that connects you to your true yearnings.

Most of us veer off our divine path as our minds take control of our lives. However, periodically your higher self may assert itself and open the doorway back to your truth. You have the choice in these moments to return to what you were always meant to be or to continue your existing path. This is your choice and no one else can make it for you.

My second divorce and all that it entailed was my big 'shunt' back onto my divine path, for the first time since my early childhood. I heard my heart and turned perceived disaster into a whole new direction. I'm proud of that.

The Arc can be a rainbow in your life connecting you to the mystical pot of gold you have not yet been able to discover, because you have been looking in the wrong place. You have been looking outside of yourself for the precious gifts in life.

You are the gift. The gold is inside your heart – the heart you may have been ignoring for much of your life. As wisdom is the creator of wealth, when you find this pot of gold inside you, your potential to create abundance of all kinds in your life will explode. You won't have to drill or mine it. You will know that you can manifest a beautiful life, but you will not need it to be perceived by others as successful, for you will be in your light, regardless of what you achieve. You will start to do things for the sheer enjoyment and pleasure of living, not to impress anyone or have anything. Judgement of yourself and others becomes a thing of your past. This is a level of freedom and sovereignty you will not want to miss.

You can use the Arc to expand, then the Arc to explore. It works in all that you do because it represents a new way of living and being. You become the human that is both being and doing, not the human that is just blindly doing. In fact, you will be the light and do at the speed of light. How could you not?

It is your bridge between your wonderful future of untold possibilities, and your past, which may contain a host of known and repeating probabilities.

It is akin to a rocket ship escaping the forces of gravity as it leaves the stratosphere of our great planet. Our consciousness enters the uncharted realms of the universe – a universe that it is very much connected to already. And it takes a trajectory to remembering where it has always been capable of going, for in spirit it has been there before and never truly left.

When you die, you will remember your ability to be one with all there is in this universe. But why not remember it now and let the great mysteries that you already are, come forth in presence.

It's time to escape the 3D information loop that keeps you mired in old ways of thinking, and in resistance to transformation that can take you to new definitions of more. Why not tune into the universal connection that exists inside you and is waiting to take you to where you are truly meant to be – in a divine place?

Phase 9 can take you past the process of arising. In this energy you have arisen. You have increased your vibration so that your true self can burst forth. You feel more fulfilled for you are fully-filled with love and light. Entering your light can only happen once you enter the vibration of love. This is where you will be in Phase 9.

In the first eight phases, you are moving through pain and closer to the truth. In Phase 9, you go above the pain and transcended it to become what God intended – the universal creator. Now you are able to participate in life in this extraordinary way.

Here lies your holy grail. You no longer need to be on that quest to find it. With the support of God, you are HOME in your own heart.

Expansion is forever so what arises from here has endless possibilities for you in your life. Universal love will open you up to infinite intelligence and an endless array of new beginnings and energies that are unique to you. And all because you decided to face your pain and illusions, and adopt a new way of living your life – one steeped in love and truth.

Is Phase 9 the End?

As I write this book, I am experiencing the wonderful benefits of Phase

9 of the Arc. Does this mean it is the end of all the phases that are possible?

I believe not, because that would not be consistent with the ever-expanding nature of the paradigms we exist within, and the universe's unlimited potential. However, this is all I can validly explain to my readers at this point. To go further would be unfounded speculation on my behalf.

As my life unfolds, I will certainly bring to readers any further insights that come into my periphery, either as later editions of this book, or in the form of additional books.

As for moving through the respective phases of the Arc, please remember that it is not a race. It's more like a memory test. The time it takes you to traverse this bridge and emerge as a new you is impossible to determine in advance. The main thing is that you start to take the steps and begin to unhook yourself from the paradigms of fear and suffering you have most likely been addicted to, perhaps for centuries.

The Arc can help you to align with the vibration of universal love. From this frequency, you can then be catapulted into the light and other higher energies, if this is your universal destiny.

The chapters that follow give you greater insights into key areas that will assist your journey into the magical duality that the Arc can illuminate – the duality of the physical and metaphysical that you already ARE.

You've got this, and you are starting to remember why!

CHAPTER 13

A Case Study of Unlearning

Exploring My Experiences Further

I mentioned that, in my own awakening journey, there were some critical matters I had to come to terms with to further my understanding and knowing of the real me.

My path has been one of great personal transformation over a nine-year period so far. I have been highly devoted to my self-discovery and have spent at least two hours a day on my unfolding, sometimes more. I have recorded every lift and realisation in bound journal books for my future reference, and to assist with my writings. At last count I had filled 55 journal books with my learnings. I have loved every minute of it, but I appreciate that readers will have different levels of time and energy that they can and will want to dedicate to their own journey.

My commitment to my expansion has mattered to me deeply because I really wanted to improve my experiences of life, which had at times been less than ideal.

My experiences have followed a series of different phases, which to date have allowed me to assimilate the high-level patterns of the Arc set out in earlier chapters.

Now I wish to offer you another lens, a more functional way of viewing my passage to higher consciousness. Remember this is my path only. We are all unique, so no two paths are the same.

I experienced:

- *Mental Phases*
  Where:
    o *I was overwhelmed by my pain, including my decision to face it, own it and tolerate it no longer.*
    o *I worked with a psychologist on my mental health.*
    o *I used mentors to strengthen my mind/personality, life/executive coach.*
    o *I learned to assess the source of my own pain and emotionalise it (i.e. releasing).*
    o *I considered my own belief structures in detail, working to find my limited subconscious beliefs and change them with my mind.*
    o *I started journaling my experiences to take my mind on the journey of discovery.*

- *Metaphysical Experiences/Phases*
  Where:
    o *Psychic experiences triggered my curiosity in the metaphysical realm.*
    o *Channelling universal wisdom sessions occurred.*
    o *I read books on the metaphysical.*
    o *I explored modalities linked to the metaphysical, including Tantra.*
    o *I had spiritual mentoring with wise individuals.*
    o *I experienced etheric connections through more evolved people, including psychics and my own direct experiences.*
    o *I visited sacred sites across the world to restate karma and enhance my self-awareness levels.*
    o *I adapted spiritual concepts to my thinking and belief structures.*

- o *I graduated as a Master of Reiki practices.*
- o *I activated my Merkabah. I discuss this later in the book, for knowledge of it is rare.*
- o *I had experiences of being omni-present.*
- o *I had direct involvement with spirits and other beings, every day. These remain active.*

- *Physical Embodiment Phases*
  Where:
  - o *Full activation of the Kundalini energy (i.e. life force) occurred inside me – at will, to eliminate energetic blockages and embodied emotions. This involved the use of kundalini yoga and activation specialists.*
  - o *Cellular shifting intensified as my awareness grew.*
  - o *Heightened awareness of synchronicity allowed me to move from understanding to knowing, through full interactions with events that unfolded.*
  - o *Exploration of the link between my physical pain and diseases, and the belief structures I held onto, allowed for healings to take place.*
  - o *I learned to physically heal myself by combining physical, medical opportunities and metaphysical energies.*

- *Transcendence Phases*
  Where:
  - o *My heart, mind, and body processed new levels of awareness instantly.*
  - o *I experienced enhanced awareness of the importance of my energy field and its link to my wholeness.*
  - o *I worked on the elimination of 'past life' karmas trapped in my energetic field and became ready to release them with a highly qualified energy field specialist. I then learned to do this myself.*

- o *Restoration of my energy field, with the same specialist, repaired damage done in this and concurrent lives.*
- o *I experienced alchemic shifts within my body.*

- *Activation Phases in Presence*
  Where:
  - o *I learned to overcome and process pain instantly in presence.*
  - o *Greater use of telepathy enabled me to communicate directly with others.*
  - o *I enjoyed feeling my own self-love (buzz) inside me.*
  - o *I allowed this love to expand into universal love and light.*
  - o *I experienced becoming universal vibrations, not just feeling and exploring them through intention.*
  - o *I became capable of manifestation through my soul connection.*
  - o *I learned to communicate with the souls of others and merge my energy fields with theirs (as appropriate).*
  - o *I experienced the dark night of the soul process, which I discuss further in this book. This altered the true meaning of fulfilment that I had applied to my life and allowed my true self to start to arise more fully. This process allows the ego to finally get out of the way and allow the creator within you to take centre stage. From here, the experience of becoming your light is possible.*

My path to higher awareness is truly not as linear as it may appear above. Several of these phases overlapped and continued concurrently at times.

My path has unfolded and transformed the essence of me, while simultaneously transforming and evolving with me. It started out being mainly mental, and this was extremely limiting, because my mind was trying to be the owner and controller of a process way beyond its comprehension. It morphed over time to be more energetic, metaphysical, and physical than mental, as I gradually reversed my way of being.

It eventually became more wholistic and more automatic.

To go deeply down the self-awareness path, requires us to give up our mental control of ourselves. It needs us to relax, feel, let go, to surrender, and allow our feelings to act as the gateway to our truths. Our egos must dissolve. This, from my experience, is a difficult concept to put into practice. The mind, body and spirit all need to interact to advance our consciousness, but their respective roles are inverse to the way most of us inherently live in the normal world.

Typically, human beings think then act. Feelings are often not accessed. More advanced human beings feel first, consider why they feel this way with reference to their beliefs, then take appropriate thoughts and actions. This is the essence of consciousness and is the embodied in the Arc.

With the help of my wonderful mentors, I worked my way down my path, sometimes faltering and sometimes feeling like I was going backwards, but always remaining committed to the ever-evolving process I was gradually remembering.

I made mistakes and I'm sure I could have got to where I am faster and with less discomfort had I been of a higher consciousness at the start. However, this is a nebulous concept in truth, because I was who and what I was. I did my best with total commitment to my unfolding. I therefore followed the path I needed to follow.

I learned my lessons the hard way, and now stand ready to show others an easier route – if they are ready! I had to remember the Arc through trial and error, assisted by the metaphysical realm. Despite having no exposure to it for the first 53 years of my life, I accepted it because in my case my experiences made it indisputable. I began to experience its direct involvement in my life, and to date have had hundreds of major metaphysical experiences. Again, this is not a badge of honour, just my own reality.

You may not experience these types of opportunities, but it does not mean you are not being supported by universal energies. You may not be able to see, feel or hear them like I can, yet; but it matters not. It doesn't mean it is not present or happening. Frankly it is no matter what you think. We simply experience what we are ready to experience.

Below are some of the key elements I needed to encounter, in addition to opening to my pain.

Letting Go of Habits and Addictions

I have not been addicted to the more common addictions in life, like gambling, drugs and alcohol, because the strict standards imposed by my mother growing up led me away from their clutches. I'm grateful to her from that. I have also always had strong will power; I had to, to get through my muscular disease issues and emotional stumbles. So, common addictions have not impacted how I dealt with pain in my life.

However, many other addictions did impact me.

Some of these were founded in my core beliefs, such as my propensity to focus too much on achieving goals, and not so much on developing relationships and doing things perfectly.

I was also addicted to time because I was always obsessed with doing, doing, doing. I found it hard to stop and relax and be present in my body. I was often thinking of future or past events, rather than being present in now moments.

I was also addicted to storytelling. I would make assumptions about the circumstances I was in, or what others were thinking. My mind thought it could tell the future or had the right to be righteous. My awareness of these traits has helped me to alter them.

I also had an addiction to suffering and giving more to others than I expected to receive.

Consequently, after all the work I have done to find my truths in life and let go of my habits and addictions, I am intolerant of anything that is not true or in integrity!

Identifying My Limiting Beliefs

We all have hundreds of unhealthy beliefs that keep us from fully enjoying our lives. I covered these in depth in my book *Where Your Happiness Hides*. Some of these beliefs arise from society, some from childhood experiences, some from unique experiences, and some from experiences in other lives.

Whatever the cause, I needed to face them all, understand and feel them, before releasing them.

When I started my awakening, I had many years of conditioning to discover and hundreds of years of karma to overcome. I began by looking back at any memories in my life that conjured up the energy of failure. This was fertile ground for it exposed experiences where I had self-destructed or sustained unexpected losses. By seeing patterns in my life, I was able to detect the limiting beliefs I had carried, then grieve and misstate the energy I held around those issues.

As I progressed, I witnessed limiting beliefs in my current life and was able to apply the Arc to dissolve them into higher consciousness, instantly.

Some limiting beliefs took multiple attempts to restate, because when I first commenced my journey, I was too 'in my head' and not sufficiently in my wholeness to process them fully.

When I attained a higher level of awareness and vibration, I discovered the process of transcendence, and this made my restatement and releasing process far more efficient and effective.

As the Arc points out, a revised belief is not embodied until it understood, known, experienced and overcome. The pain of a limiting belief is normally needed to be felt for you to fully comprehend how it has depreciated your life's experiences.

Sometimes the experiences I needed to be challenged by to alter my energies took time to arise, and sometimes I was unsuccessful when I faced them in the first instance, such that I reintroduced the old belief structures and needed to challenge myself again and again. But I never gave up on my desire to release them.

Some of my limiting beliefs were derived from past lives and were therefore karmic in nature. Although some of them had created similar patterns in this life, I initially needed the assistance of much more aware people than me, with more proficient metaphysical abilities, to identify and help me release them. I found this to be highly entertaining because of the stories that arose. However, these releases were also difficult to attain at times because they required deep personal enquiry, and my soul would not release me from the karmic belief patters until I had a 100% understanding of their importance to my learning and could articulate it fully.

Examples of the core limiting beliefs that I held included beliefs like:

- *I am not lovable unless I make lots of money.*
- *I must suffer to get what I want in life.*
- *Money is more important than love.*
- *I must win at all costs.*
- *I am not as good looking or valuable as other men.*
- *Love must be controlled or else it will abandon me.*

It took me years to identify all these limiting self-beliefs. As time went by, I discovered that I did not need to hunt these down. All I needed to do was ask spirits to show me the beliefs that were holding me back, and they began to show themselves to me automatically. I just needed to witness them and respond consciously and with feeling and integrity.

Your soul knows when you are ready to release a limiting belief.

To get ahead of this divine process is not advisable, and probably the biggest lesson I learned from my journey thus far.

Releasing My Unhealthy Validations

Our ego does its best in our lives to protect our reputations and to project a positive image on our behalf, so that we feel valued, validated, and lovable. This leads us to have certain things we rely upon to help us feel valid in the eyes of others. It is without doubt a form of delusion, because as a child of God, or the universe, we can never be anything other than valid.

I encountered several matters that I clung to, to feel validated in life. These included:

- *Winning anything I took part in, including sports.*
- *Having a big house so I appeared to be successful to friends and family.*
- *Being in a successful romantic relationship.*
- *Always being in control of my emotions.*
- *Being fit, so I looked more lovable.*
- *Having an active sex life within the bounds of my romantic relationships.*

Most of my validations were conditioned into me by society. This made it easy to forgive myself for having them. They are essentially fears – 'if this does not occur, I am not lovable' is the typical source of all validations.

As I worked through my pain and limiting beliefs, I was able to systematically expose and release these validations. I now feel valid no matter what circumstances I face, for I know I am complete within myself. Nothing outside of me can therefore complete me. These validations were in place because of certain beliefs I held. They are closely linked.

Along my journey, the universe systematically stripped me of the most potent things that validated me, to show me through the experience of pain, that they truly could never define the true me. This, of course, was very painful to go through, but was the reality of the expansionary path that I chose in this life.

Releasing New Sources of Pain

Over time, I was able to release the core pains and scars that I carried from my past experiences. This I am proud of and grateful for. However, I soon discovered that I could not rest on my laurels. I was still alive and involved in life's circumstances, so I was still generating positive and negative experiences and emotions in every new day.

This is where I discovered that, to stay relatively pain-free and in a place of happiness, I needed to process pain and disappointment the moment that I became aware of them. I could not wait and carry the scars for long because I felt disturbed when my energy field was out of sync. I felt pain in my body as well. The higher your vibration rises the less you can tolerate density and it starts to weigh heavily on your feelings when they are unresolved.

In my place of higher vibration, I now find that I am more prone to speak my truth to others on a timely basis to resolve issues than ever before, and to release the emotions relating to pain far more quickly. If I have a physical problem, I attend to it fast with doctors, and by considering my personal contributions to that pain.

My acceptance of suffering has effectively diminished, and my addiction is now to truth happiness, and integrity, rather than pain.

I have also become more familiar in expressing my emotions in front of other people, including family and friends. There is a core understanding in me that relationships exist to help us find our own truths, and to witness ourselves with greater clarity. They are a wonderful mirror into our selves.

Other people, therefore, deserve our expression of truth with compassion on a timely basis. I wasn't always good at this. The suppression or distortion of truth becomes less tolerable as we journey to higher levels of self-awareness.

Exiting Toxic Relationships

Many of us are prone to accept and continue to be in relationships that are not in our best interests or may be somewhat toxic for us. *I have done this many times in my life.*

We are often drawn to people who can provide us with a mirror into our own selves. There are often lessons to be learned about ourselves from interacting with these people, but once these lessons are seen and felt, it is important that we take the most appropriate action for our own well-being and happiness. This can include no longer interacting with these people, although I understand how difficult and painful it can be to end close relationships, particularly in family situations.

I've been there and done that and endured much pain as a result. My relationship with my mother, for example, was tumultuous as I matured, and for a number of years I kept my distance from her somewhat controlling patterns. Eventually, forgiveness descended into this relationship. This took me a lot of inner work to achieve.

It doesn't mean you need to hate or disregard these people. In fact, you can continue to love them. However, it's important that in the process of assessing the relationship that you truly value yourself. You are here to live your life for you, and not live your life for the sake of others.

In a sense, the giver often attracts the taker in relationships. This is the natural mirror at play, and is intended to reveal to both parties their conditioned predilections. In its extreme form, an anxious or empathic lover will often attract a narcissistic or dismissive individual into a romantic relationship. There is often an imbalance that needs to be seen and grown through; but unless both individuals are prepared to learn and grow together, and on their own, this form of contrast can prove too hard to endure for both parties.

There is much literature in books and on the internet about relating styles, but the bottom line is that your sense of self may not be served by devoting your time and energies to individuals who do not contribute to your happiness and sense of fulfilment if they are unwilling to change and compromise.

I had a pattern of staying in relationships that did not truly serve me for far too long. In some of these relationships, I felt used and disrespected, but I was driven too strongly by my aversion to failure, which included romantic relationships, career arrangements and friendships.

I consider myself to be a kind and giving person, but what realised in the end was that this propensity was not always a badge of honour and often led me to a form of self-deprecation. I had developed people-pleasing tendencies that needed to be seen and faced. I always wanted to be the saviour of others to my own detriment. This took me many years to recognise and act upon.

Essentially, I had a lack of self-worth, and this was keeping me in toxic relationships that I did not enjoy. Again, my inner reality became my outer reality. Now that my conscious awareness is higher, I have become far more discerning about the people with whom I spent my life.

I know that, essentially, there is love between us all at a metaphysical level; but a person's level of self-awareness, strength of ego and depth of conditioning can mean a mismatch in the physical world with others, and it may not be in our interests to participate with that.

Applying the Arc to your conscious awareness can help you to expand, and in turn lead you to your own tribe of people with aligned ways of being, thinking and living. And the composition of your tribe will change over your lifetime as you continue to evolve.

Mine certainly has.

The Dreaded Spiritual Ego

As you expand and grow by applying consciousness to gain awareness, there is a trap you are more than likely to fall into. It is a deep trap that is hard to get out of for it is hard to witness. This is created by what is called the spiritual ego.

As we become more aware and advanced in consciousness, our ego starts to find a new avenue of expression. With less normal egoic junk to express, it turns its attention to your new founded awareness and claims it as a mark of superiority and achievement.

Your newfound spiritual awareness effectively becomes a badge of honour to your ego. It declares that you are ahead of, and therefore superior to, less self-aware people. To do this, it is forming judgements that it has no right to make or ability to truly do. A person's level of awareness varies in each lifetime and is fundamentally between them and their soul. No one has the right to rank others on any grounds for we are all getting what we need and living the life that we need.

It is easy to observe how many spiritually aware people often change their core habits in the face of their newfound spiritual egos and perceived achievements. They may start to dress differently to the rest of society, to signify that they now identify with a more spiritual subset of people. Happy pants become just a new form of uniform, like a suit has historically been in the business world. Some change their names to indicate that they have arisen to new heights, and some may change where they live, to retreat from a world with which they now find great fault.

There are limitations in normal life that are derived from commonly held conditioned belief structures. However, to judge this and not accept others or life as it is, is tantamount to playing God. It is naïve to think that we are above what is, for we are a part and connected to the great tapestry of life and the universe as it unfolds.

As I often say God has the plan, we do not need our own. The truth is we wrote our own life plan before birth, then we were born and out of ignorance we try and write it again, rather than access the divine one already sitting in the Akashic Records with our soul's agreement.

I entertained the dreaded spiritual ego in my life for a period until I witnessed its presence. It is insidious and difficult to avoid.

As you venture through the Arc, you may yourself come face-to-face with it. I would be surprised if you don't.

The spiritual ego also has a close 'cousin' called spiritual avoidance. When pain arises, the spiritual avoider goes to meditation, or some other practice, to escape their pain. Escaping pain can mask it or even take it out of our conscious thoughts temporarily. However, the universe is sure to bring us back into a collision with that pain at some point, so that we again have the opportunity to open to it and learn from its wisdom.

Universal love is the only source of truth in this world. Returning to our natural state as universal love gives us unparalleled access to this truth, and the fastest way to this wonderful place is to evolve through unlearning. Once we unlearn what we are not, our souls can remind us of what we really are.

Why not unlearn your way to the mysteries that lie within you!

CHAPTER 14

Overcoming Physical Pain

Are You the Architect of Your Own Pain?

If you are reading this book and pondering the topic of loving your pain away, I'm sure you have probably begun to consider how this principle can possibly apply to physical pain in your body.

Emotional pain, of course, can be more transient, and you should have more control over it once you find the pathway to your soul, because it is often related to stress.

However, I am a walking, talking example of how physical pain can be overcome when you apply the principles espoused in this book, as long as it is derived from your own limiting beliefs and is not purely physical.

Let me tell you my story of debilitating pain, and then I will outline the wisdom that flowed to me from this experience. It is not wisdom you will hear from many mainstream doctors in the Western world, because they mainly work with the physicality of your body, not your belief structures that impact upon them. Some holistic practitioners may, however, align with my views, such as Reiki practitioners, acupuncturists, Chinese doctors and other energy-based healers.

At the age of 19, I developed a muscular disorder that, according to doctors, had no name and no cure. It was not until 14 years later that it was diagnosed and given a name by the only doctor in the world who reportedly treated it. In this time, different treatments were recommended and tried by me, but none of them were successful.

My muscle disorder caused me great pain and was to last for nearly 40 years. The primary symptom I endured in this terrible period was muscle cramping through my whole body, day and night. Sleep was my only real escape. Otherwise, it never let up.

Other main symptoms I endured included:

- *A locking jaw that continuously dislocated because of the cramps around the base of my skull and in my head. This would occur about 15 times a minute, and sometimes I could not eat because my jaw was jammed shut, and I needed the help of a dentist to open it, particularly in the mornings after I had slept.*
- *Itchy skin, but with no rash, because my nervous system was working overtime to deal with my muscular problems.*
- *Migraine headaches most days of the week that required me to seek solitude. These typically occurred in the evenings after my day at work.*
- *Constant dizziness and loss of balance.*
- *Bouts of asthma because of the muscle pressure around my lungs. I was a strong athlete growing up and was told by one doctor that I had massive lung capacity, so to end up with asthma for an extended period was difficult.*
- *Bad neck and back pain up and down my spine because the muscle spasms were putting pressure on the discs in my back. This required constant visits to my chiropractor, but relief was normally only short lived.*
- *Muscle spasms around my neck and head, like ticks that others endure in Tourette's Syndrome, which were not only uncomfortable but also embarrassing to endure.*
- *Constriction in my body associated with the cramping and shortening of muscles that made playing sports more difficult.*

- *I displaced a disk in my neck at one stage because of my neck muscle pressure, and my arm withered away until it recovered about three months later.*

I was told that the muscle cramps would eventually harm other aspects of my body, including my eyes and heart, because they were reliant on muscular proficiency to operate properly. It was a race against time, because my doctor believed I would eventually sustain heart attacks if effective treatments were not found, because the heart is a muscle that pumps blood. It would eventually seize up.

Fortunately, this did not occur, but on his advice, I swam regularly to keep my body in good shape so I could limit the impacts of the muscle cramping.

To try and solve my problems, I visited a myriad of doctors and specialists including:

- *Physiotherapists,*
- *Chiropractors,*
- *Dentists and orthodontists,*
- *Heart specialists,*
- *Orthopaedic surgeons,*
- *Pain management experts,*
- *Alexander technique specialists,*
- *Musculoskeletal podiatrists, and*
- *An acupuncturist.*

The list goes on. The most effective treatments came from dental specialists, because through the treatment of my teeth they were able to alter the muscle relationships around my jaw and release some of the physical tension and cramps I had in this area of my body. However, this course of treatment saw me have braces twice on my teeth, and eventually led me to replace 10 of my teeth with dental crowns, when it became apparent that the braces could not sufficiently cure the muscular disorders.

All up, this disease was a problem I would not wish upon my worst enemy. It made my life extremely painful and difficult for many years and distracted me from activities I wanted to pursue. I never considered suicide, but there were times when I thought death would have been an easier outcome.

The cure for this terrible disease came, though, when I owned it as a part of me. Until I did this, I effectively tried to hide and suppress it in my life, because I did not want others to judge me as not good enough or flawed. I was already emotionally impacted by the pain, and I had already judged myself harshly as a result.

I also refused to take drugs or drink alcohol to overcome my pain, because something inside me told me that would be tantamount to giving in to the disease. I refused to submit to it, choosing to separate myself from it as best I could.

Later in my life, however, I had a breakthrough that enabled me to overcome the disease. And it all came when I applied consciousness to my physical pain.

What I discovered, as I followed my path to higher awareness, was that I was the architect of the disease. Yes, it existed in physical terms, but I had manifested it out of deep insecurities and stress. As I wrote in my book Where Your Happiness Hides, *the fact that I was not living, as my true self, created the stress that led to the disease. I was out of alignment with my truth, and doing too many things I did not love. I wasn't really enjoying my life and I was fundamentally unhappy and tolerating aspects of my life. In short, I was living my life hoping to find happiness without truly connecting to the disease inside me. Self-love was absent.*

The first time I ever detected the disease was on the first day I started my career as a chartered accountant. This was a clue that I was incapable of linking to my self-esteem until I reached my later years. I was in a career I did not really like, and my soul was warning me that I could still rechoose my career direction. I ignored it out of conditioned thinking. Besides, I was in a job that, with the help of others, my mind had chosen, not my heart.

By not opening to my pain, other than through doctors, and effectively hiding it from others, I allowed the source of the disease to gather intensity. My life got busier and more complex as I got married, had children, and advanced up through the ranks in my career. I was grateful for the things I had in life, but the relentless obligations and lack of fun led me to increasing levels of misalignment and stress. I had given up most of my hobbies and fun activities to devote to family and making money to support them. I did this willingly because I loved them.

When my consciousness journey started to unfold and advance, I learned to enquire and tune into my emotional pain to solve it and gain higher levels of conscious awareness. Then I realised I could do this same process with my physical pain.

Each time, the pain in my back, neck, jaw, or other bodily areas, intensified with cramping, I would simply ask my heart what I was meant to be aware of or change in this situation, and what wisdom would help me gain relief. And I got answers.

Each response made me question certain beliefs, and then I applied the Arc further to help me transcend them. Each time I altered my beliefs and actions I would receive further relief from the pain.

It was clear. My pain was my indicator that I needed to change some things, and when I did what was required, the pain would leave me in peace until the next indicator arose. Gradually by applying this approach, I defeated the disease.

Now I know that, if symptoms of the disease ever appear again, even in a mild form, I have slipped back into old habits and my body is warning me that a course correction is required.

By defeating this disease, I got to witness the strength and resilience that lies within me. I am now very proud of this. However, I must accept the reality that my health was unknowingly wrecked by my own illusions and ignorance for many years.

I have used this practice now many times on other physical ailments with the same success. I might still visit a doctor, but I know that they will probably only be able to treat the symptoms of a disease. The true source of the symptoms may well have its origin in my beliefs and life choices.

The Wholeness of Physical Pain

In our Western culture, we tend to look at the physical pain we experience and ascribe it to a physical cause only. But we are energy as well as matter and, therefore, both must be looked at to attain a fast effective healing.

Other more wholistic healing practices seem to be more conscious in the way they treat pain because they look beyond the physical.

Acupuncture and Chinese medicine practitioners have given me wonderful healings that Western medicine consultations could not seemingly give me.

For example, I was told by a highly respected cardiologist, who treated me for years, that I was born with an unusual heart rhythm that included an extra heartbeat. This I was told was incurable.

My acupuncturist healed it within two minutes, because he somehow linked the problem to the flow of energy through my body.

By denying or delaying the impact of our own choices and beliefs on our bodies, we deny ourselves the chance to influence our own physical healing.

Of course, if you get injured in a physical accident or are impacted by a genetic issue, there will be pain that our minds have not influenced.

But for many diseases we do naïvely divorce ourselves from our pain, like I did all those years ago, and miss out on healing we could initiate for ourselves. Such pain is always a signpost. The difficulty is discovering what the signpost is pointing to, which may not be clear.

It may well be reflecting the residual of an old injury, particularly if the problem is not healed or treated. Whenever there is a wound or pain of any kind, be it physical or emotional, it is energetically advantageous to treat it as soon as possible so that there are far fewer residual problems later.

When such a pain remains unresolved, it will present itself to us again and again. Frankly that is its job. All it is doing is asking us for healing. Of course, our medical systems may not support this fast healing due to lack of resources or funding, and this is a major problem in many nations. This is why we see systemic issues with pain that have not been dealt with properly or fast enough. They continue to arise for clearing.

This also applies to issues arising in so-called past lives, which continue to influence our current energies and mindsets.

The challenge is identifying where the signpost of pain is pointing. What healing does it require?

Until we find the true source of our pain it will continue to repeat itself. The risk is that our bodies adapt to the ongoing circumstances of the pain and effectively make the situation worse.

When my muscular disease afflicted my life, I could not treat it physically because it had no name or known cure. The doctors were stumped. If I had faced its emotional source earlier, I could have overcome it earlier. Instead, the disease impacted on other parts of my life in detrimental ways. It became a part of me and the way I lived, because I did not have the consciousness to deal with it early on in my life. I forgive myself for this, for I did the best I could do.

The more awareness we can bring to the root cause of any pain, the greater likelihood we will have of healing it permanently. If we never find that awareness, we can take the energetic source of the issue to our graves. This is where you can use the Arc to bring the totality of your pain into your conscious receptivity. Logical or physical assessments will only get you so far and may never lead you to the truth.

We should consider all relevant aspects of a physical experience leading to pain to ensure that we have also treated the emotional impacts of that event.

At the age of five, I was beaten up by four teenage boys on my way home from kindergarten. I was thrown against a barb wire fence and brutally punched, and I still carry the scars on my legs from this event. I was physically treated in hospital after the attack, and I was asked to confront my attackers at their homes so they could apologise.

What no one, including me, thought about was the emotional scars I would carry because of this attack. I therefore suppressed the emotional scars.

In my 60s, I finally faced the emotional pain of this harrowing ordeal alone. I relived what I experienced in graphic detail and sobbed intensely. I realised that it had caused me to lose trust in people.

I got stitches and an apology within days, but my psychology was clearly disturbed for much of my life because I had suppressed it.

The universe does not want to see you in pain. It wants you to learn and expand through experiences, and return to the knowing of what you truly are – pure love living a physical life through conscious awareness with a birthright to be happy. That's one of the core reasons you have chosen to be alive on Earth now.

The universe will provide you with the means to release the pain of your wounds back into totality – all you have to do is go to the love that is beneath the pain and ask for its release in the face of higher awareness – on a timely basis if possible. Pain in the human experience is otherwise very solitary because we normally believe in the concept of separation or individuation.

I had the great privilege of healing cancer in my head and ears by following this belief or process. This was minor cancer. I recognise that I did not have a major cancer illness like I know others have had to endure. My doctor to this day remains confused that the cancer was defeated without specialist medical attention.

In truth, I did not heal it; the universe did at my request, and with my cooperation and growing self-awareness. I used my Reiki capabilities and my communion with God to co-create this outcome.

I also used this process to overcome Covid when it arose in my body a few times. Twenty minutes of meditation and it was gone every time. No vaccinations needed.

Clearing pain in our physical bodies is very challenging because we believe that we need to go out there to doctors to get help, because we are defenceless otherwise. Investigating the root cause of any pain, including physical pain, is an integral step to healing. Going inward to find the root cause in terms of our beliefs and behaviours can expediate the healing process, as can aligning with the life force within us. And there are people around us who can also help with this endeavour.

I worked with a woman who did this kind of work through a modality known as Body Talk. She helped me greatly by exposing the links between my beliefs and a number of ailments I carried.

Is this more conscious healing a form of miracle healing? Yes and no!

Mankind would call this kind of healing a miracle because it refuses to accept that it is possible, unless carried out by a pure being like Jesus Christ. However, the truth is: it is a natural remedy that's available to us all when we simply believe in the powerful vibration of love, we are all connected to. After all, love has the most potent vibration in the universe and is the source of all creation.

I have used it multiple times and I'm no saint, just a normal human being like you, who has mastered the Arc and combined it with modern medicines! In this way, the metaphysical and physical have come together to restore my health. This mirrors the very way that we live – in both realms.

Honouring Your Physical Indicators

One of the key physical factors I discovered as I applied the Arc, was that I have certain recurring indicators in my body that have become my soul's personal messengers that I have fallen back to ego and fear. These indicators arose at different points of my evolution. My soul uses them to tell me in no uncertain terms that change is needed urgently, either in what I am believing, thinking, or doing.

I have three at present, which are:

- *My left knee seizes up when I enter an environment where I am either overstating or understating my self-worth, relative to others. I have trouble walking until I stop and sit with the pain and listen to its wisdom. Once I hear its message and make the right mental adjustments, the pain goes away instantly.*
- *My left hand, and particularly my left thumb, locks up and aches when I enter an environment that stimulates some form of grief from my past that I have yet to fully transcend. Again, as soon as I witness the issue and restate my beliefs, the hand frees up and becomes pain free.*
- *My right neck muscles tighten and can lock up when I step out of alignment with my true desires and intentions in any situation and have therefore started to align with what others want me to do or be, rather than what I want to do or be. It points me to compromises I truly did not want to make, so I can correct them.*

It is much cheaper and faster when these three indicators arise to tune into my pain, rather than rush off to a doctor or physiotherapist. It usually only takes minutes to fix the issues.

This is a natural form of healing that has sustainable benefits for the way I live my life, and it also brings me higher awareness at the same time.

I may encounter new indicators as I age.

My soul will determine this. My job is to listen and allow it to lead me forward.

Loving Your Body

One of the key things I came to understand from applying a more conscious approach to healing was that I needed to reverse my perspectives on my body and its relationship to my egocentric mind.

When I suffered through my many years of intense pain with my debilitating muscle disorder, I blamed my body for the pain and torment it was seemingly creating for me. I know that it lowered my self-esteem substantially, because I thought that my body was deeply flawed and not good enough. I felt life had let me down.

I eventually came to see that it was the reverse.

My limited mind was creating unwanted circumstances in my life. What my body was doing through its wisdom, was showing my mind how to solve the pain. It was a source of higher intelligence I did not tune into until I was in my 50s. The body was my wise indicator and informant, and was flashing red, until I stopped believing it was at fault.

Next time you feel pain in your body, remember that it is, in many cases, wisdom coming from your soul and intended for your mind. The body is the connector between your soul and your mind. It is the source of all feeling and wants to be heard.

Your body was selected for you by your soul before you were born. The truth is you chose it. It is therefore, the perfect body to bring you the experiences and learnings you were meant to have in this life, not the ones your ego thinks you were meant to have.

It will also attract the primary partners you are meant to be with in this incarnation. These key partners and the relationships you will share with them are intended and will arise in divine timing.

Not everyone will love your body and how it looks, but the main person who needs to, and can love it, is you. It's just a new belief away.

So next time you are standing in front of a mirror and feeling underwhelmed, or experiencing a rejection from someone who does not find you attractive, remember all the wonderful wisdom and positives that your body has brought into your life. Without the body you have, you would not be here today having the experiences you hold dear.

Love your body and care for it because it matters, and is enough, just like you are in every way.

Comparisons to the bodies owned by others are truly meaningless, for they are walking a different path to you, and chose the right body to make their individual journey possible. It was a gift from the universe, not a problem or masterpiece created by your parents. They just supplied the DNA you needed to make your body possible.

With so many body image issues causing unhappiness in this world, the deep understanding that everyone chose the body they live within, for deep purpose, could surely lower many mental health conditions we witness today, particularly among younger people who are often forced to be quite image conscious by societal conditioning. This is not their fault.

Again, pain management could be replaced and eliminated for many, through the power of greater conscious awareness, including a closer understanding of our belief structures and the reality of choice.

Healing Through the Frequency of Love

In advanced stages of your alignment with the frequency of love, self-healing capabilities arise as you find a greater equilibrium within yourself.

You are truly immersed in the frequency of love. It is inside you and all around you. There is pure love in the air we breathe, the sunlight that warms us, the water we drink, bathe and swim within, the soil we walk upon and the universal energies that we continually interact with. These energies can heal us when we commune with it, for they possess the power of love. Of course, mankind can bring toxicity to nature as it does within its own energy fields and bodies, in turn diluting its beneficial qualities temporarily with pollution.

Let us take the air we breathe as an example. It is so beneficial to your physical experience to allow yourself the deep resonance of love to enter the bloodstream through your breath. It is possible to open to the experience of feeling the frequency of this love begin to circulate through your body as your heart pumps your blood throughout your veins. This is why so many people do breathwork as a spiritual modality.

However, what they may not understand is that the cleansing qualities of love are present when they exhale and inhale every breath. They don't need to do it once a month in a group setting to achieve healings. You can do it wherever you are, all day long.

When you include and begin to experiment with the sensation of breathing in love, you begin to experience extraordinary sensory expansion. But this is beyond the ordinary concepts of mainstream thinking and modern Western medicine. However, this form of healing is a truly natural healing capability of any being in human form.

When you set the intention, to surrender to the frequency of love within you, and ask it to adjust or heal all that is out of alignment within you, it will harmonise what is disagreeing with your natural state of being. You mind will know what pains you have and can direct the vibrations to that part of your physicality. But if you surrender to this frequency fully, it will find its own way through your physicality. It has the capacity to heal even what you might be unaware needs healing.

This frequency of love knows you better than your mind knows you. It can take some time to penetrate the beliefs of the mind, so that it understands that there is a greater and more powerful resource than it, for all the activities you participate in, in your life. When you let the frequency of love become an aspect of your awakening, you can find a greater level of balance and equilibrium in all you do. You gradually become centred in all aspects of your life, and this is of great benefit to your body and its cellular structures.

That pain in your back or shoulder that you are conscious of, may not even originate from physical deficiencies in that part of your body, but from another body part; or it may have an emotional origin for instance, as was the case with my muscular disease.

For example, a lot of back pain originates from burden. If you tune into the awareness of the source of this burden, and make the necessary changes in your life, guess what is likely to happen to the pain?

I had chronic back pain during most of my 30s and 40s. It was so bad at times I had to use a device to pick things up from the floor. When I started to explore my self-awareness through the Arc, it vanished instantly and completely. I was its architect.

Stress will often attack a core weakness in your body, for here it can bring about the most potent awareness through pain. We feel the relayed energy most in these parts of our body, because they are less resistant and healthy.

The vibration of love understands it all and will bring the awareness of the pain to you if you tune into its wisdom. Remember this is not referring to the conditioned love we think we understand. This is the frequency of love that can only ever be known and felt – a universal energy beyond the conception of the mind.

This is a massive advantage of learning to live as pure love. Whether it's love from the sun, the ocean or in the air, nature is a healing resource that has immense power if we draw it in and tune into its incredible healing powers.

The body also has its own internal healing light that can alter our physical wellbeing, if we trust in it and allow it to do so. It's like having a medical centre within you that is constantly keeping your cellular structure healthy. No insurance needed! And you age much slower when you harness the power of this knowing. Ageing is impacted by the density of our energy fields and bodies. It is related to the passing of negative beliefs and thoughts, not the truth of love.

Humanity is obsessed with slowing down the ageing process. Love is the true answer not considered in laboratories all around the world. This is not surprising. It's hard to make money selling a 'no-thing' that is free within us all.

I never got Covid during the pandemic, despite living in a home that it often visited and was present for a number of weeks. Why? Because I harnessed the vibration of love within me, the sunlight, and my breath every day, and asked it to overcome the disease if it ever entered my body or field. A virus has a vibration just like us. However, it is no match for the power of the vibration of love.

Like everything in life your physical and metaphysical realities merge to create the whole you. This includes your health. To overcome any physical pain, it is in your best interests to seek appropriate medical advice and to *support* that with an exploration of the wisdom inherent in your pain. You never know you may be the architect of your demise!

CHAPTER 15

Ownership of Pain

Pain Consciousness, Not Management

Our world is full of people who get paid to help us manage or remove our pain. Most are well-intended and caring souls; but the reality is, the longer it takes to remove your pain, the more it can financially benefit them.

But handing them responsibility for our pain management is not just detrimental to us financially, it is detrimental to us emotionally. Pain is an indicator created within you, for the benefit of you, no one else. You are the only one on the planet it is trying to talk to. You are the only one who can feel it. By giving it to someone else to manage, we lose the possibility for new levels of self-awareness to enter our consciousness.

Sometimes pain can be shared by many because of a single event, such as a war or unexpected death; but in that collective experience, each of us will receive our own unique signal that something is not right, and something different needs to take place for us as individuals.

The source of our pain can vary in its significance; but, as a rule, the longer it is left unattended the more damage it will do to you, mentally, physically, and emotionally. It is a noose around your neck that you may be able to sever.

If you have done physical damage to your body, perhaps in an accident, the pain is probably asking you to seek medical treatment.

If your physical pain is being caused by your own worry and stress, you can use professional help to assist with the symptoms, and your own inner resources to deal with the true source of the pain which revolves around your beliefs.

If the pain relates to mental health issues, the pain is trying to tell you that you have the power within yourself to overcome the issues. Experts like psychologists or mentors, may be of great assistance in helping you to understand your pain and take steps to alleviate it. They can spark your awareness.

But the first step is to always own and love the pain, as strange as this may sound. You need to be the one who takes the steps forward and finds the awareness to rid yourself of the pain and any associated symptoms.

Pain management can imply that we have accepted that pain will be present with us for an extended period. We can wear this type of pain as a badge of honour and too easily accept its presence, particularly as we age. This is not a winning strategy.

When I presented to doctors in my early years with my debilitating muscle pain, a number of those doctors advised me to take drugs to manage my pain. I refused, because to me that was the equivalent of giving up and letting the disease win. It is not in my nature to give up, no matter how intense my pain is. I told the doctors that the disease was not going to beat me.

What I got wrong for much of the duration of my disease, was that I did not let go and surrender to the pain it was causing me, so I could harness new self-awareness levels to overcome it. I did the right thing not giving up, because to give up would have seen me enter the endless path of pain management through drug therapy.

Pain is ours, and only ever ours to own. It is a part of us. We need to honour it as it is honouring you.

Giving Up Versus Letting Go

One thing my disease and other difficult events taught me, is the fundamental difference between letting go and giving up. I wish I had understood this earlier in my life.

Letting go is an energy aligned with love and trust. It is a foundation of conscious advancement, for we are trusting that our inner sense loves us and knows what we need to do to attain peace in any situation. When we let go or surrender to a problem that is bringing us pain, we can tune into a cure. In this energy, we can listen to our pain with full integrity, through the conscious receptivity embedded in the Arc. We can then use what we hear to make the necessary changes or seek suitable assistance to overcome a problem.

Giving up is a controlling energy. It is based on ignorance and fear. When we give in our minds are saying to the universe, "I know better than you about the future and I know what to expect." Expectation is often born out of illusion. We play God when we give up, because we believe we are fully in control of our lives. What if we don't know what our future holds?

My advice with pain is not to *give up*, but to instead *let go*. Surrender to its wisdom and feel it fully, unless to do so would be debilitating of course. There may be situations where we have left the cure too late, and we lose our chance to overcome a painful problem. When it comes to pain, time is often of the essence, quite literally.

But if we can trust our essence, or energy, we can successfully mitigate or overcome many sources of pain. It is how we are naturally meant to live our lives.

My disease lasted nearly 40 years. If I had given up and not listened to its message after all that time, it would still be with me today. I'm glad I never gave up, and instead finally let go. But I should have let go much earlier!

The world needs to invest more resources into medical services so people can address their pain earlier than they do now. Perhaps less money spent on the military to inflict pain and more on health to heal it would not go astray. Radical thinking, I know!

Owning Pain Publicly

We all experience emotions. They are natural. Still, we often try to avoid expressing our pain to others for the fear that it will make us look weak, and incapable of coping with the issues in our life. Who wants to be seen as weak or in pain!

When people meet in Western cultures, we often ask, "How are you today?" with the standard answer being, "I'm good, how are you?"

We don't really want to disclose that we might be in some form of pain, as that would dispel the image of perfection that we try so hard to create. Such conversations would also probably take all day, given how much accumulated emotional pain we all carry though life!

And does anyone asking these questions really care about the answers they get?

The answer is truly: the strong ones care. The courageous ones among us have the strength to be real, to really listen to others, and to own our own pain publicly when that is appropriate. We need to encourage this.

Crying is the antitheses of this image problem. When we cry in front of others, we believe we will be deflated or condemned in their eyes. But what is more important, our happiness and health, or our image?

Crying is a natural process that takes place within us to allow energy to put in motion. It releases bad, and sometimes good, energies to allow them to move out of our bodies and our energy fields. This release normally allows the mitigation of pain to take place quite quickly. As we are doing this release, the truth of the pain can become obvious!

Thus, while it is helpful to think about the source and solution to our pain, we must understand that thoughts are not the pain itself, they are electrical impulses in our brains; so if we are in pain, it is more important to surrender to it and release it through a natural movement of energy. You won't overcome pain by thinking it away, but feeling it away is a different paradigm.

If you have ever been in a relationship that has ended painfully, like I have multiple times, it is so tempting to spend all our time rationalising the reasons why it ended, until we arrive at a logical point of wanting to be at peace. But we can never be at peace with any painful experience until we find the peace within ourselves, and this peace must be established energetically. It must be felt, not rationalised; and the process of crying is a natural gateway to this important release of feeling.

Water is highly correlated with the emotional body that exists within us, which is why being near or in water can assist us to express pain. When we cry, we release water in the form of tears. Water carries the vibration of unconditional love. So, when we cry, we are also undertaking a process that is very self-loving. It is not a process that should be judged in any other light.

In spiritual terms, waterfalls are known to enhance our ability to connect us to our true selves. This is not a myth! I have experienced it with great power myself in Samoa. Waterfalls are a physical representation of 'As Above So Below' in universal terms. Crying sets off our own inner waterfalls, allowing the fluid within us to flow over us, as tears.

Crying is not the only form of pain release. Screaming and yelling are other examples, although these may be best expressed alone, and not in public settings, for they can become offensive and intrusive to others if they are not controlled properly by the person in pain.

Isn't it time we learned to cry to our heart's content?

Owning Your Energy

As intuitive beings we all feel energy. We may not be conscious of the fact, but it is inescapable. Some people may be more intuitive than others, but no one person has a mortgage on feeling energy.

When we carry pain into a relationship or event, others will therefore feel it. We will also feel it within us. This energy not only impacts upon those unfolding circumstances but, unless it is reshaped, this energy will most likely impact our future relationships – even the relationships we have with ourselves.

Releasing pain changes your energy field, body, and mind such that it has a positive impact on the energy of any situation. But to do this we must first take ownership of both our pain, and the effect it has on others.

A Pain-Free Paradise

Once we become more experienced in using the Arc, we can start to live without any substantive pain, simply because we can view it with curiosity and face it quickly. This primarily relates to pain that is linked to our emotions and belief structures, and not pure physical pain from external events such as being hit by a bus. We can repeatedly transform ourselves, and easily return to a place of peace. This is a wonderful place to reach, and it is your birthright to be happy in this way, by processing then ultimately rejecting all forms of self-imposed suffering.

As you become more conscious, one thing you will notice is that you naturally become happier. You apply the Arc, or the version of it that works for you, to create new possibilities out of pain and your sense of self can't help but arise.

Then another issue arises in your life, and you become increasingly aware about how to deal with it and return to a place of peace. You get faster and faster at seeking relief as time goes on. Your evolution supports less tolerance for unhappiness and suffering.

What I have found is that I have become increasingly comfortable with pain and discomfort. Why? Because I know I have the tools to learn from it and dismiss it almost instantly. Pain is effectively dismissed by the self-awareness that it helps me to create. It's a natural bridge between my past losses or disruptions, and my current happiness.

In the latter phases of the Arc, you learn to hand the energies associated with learning back to the universe from whence it came. This energy has served you and can be passed back to be used by others to help them evolve. All is energy, and all is ultimately shared, for we are one.

Much of your pain is karmic, meaning it has been built up energetically from living through the density of the past on Earth. But you have the opportunity to open to it in this life and let it go now!

For someone who is naturally curious, particularly about myself, the Arc has given me a very fast escape route from pain and suffering. It can come back if I don't fully surrender to it, but each time it is diminished. There is no need to manage a pain that is wise but can also be fleeting. I love my pain to its own demise. And then I rest in peace while I am still alive.

Is it time you learned to rest in peace while you are still in human form, and not continue to wait until you pass for this wonderful state?

CHAPTER 16

Losing the Plot in Our Pain

The Fiction of our Futures and Pasts

It's important to note that we all constantly tell ourselves stories about our lives.

The stories of our futures are usually written by our egos and are normally designed to protect and promote us, for that is the core bias of the ego. These stories are often full of hope, assumption, and expectation. However, they can, and from my own experience often do, set us up for pain and suffering, for they are not steeped in truth. They are fairy tales.

Here are some examples of the type of stories we often create for ourselves:

- My partner is my one and only soul mate, we will live happily ever after.
- I'll get rich and retire by the age of 60.
- I will never get a serious disease, like others.
- After I reach the next milestone in my career, I will have more freedom and be happier.
- I will feel more secure once I have a certain amount of savings.
- A big and flash home will show others how successful I am.

I once wrote these exact stories in my own mind, with full confidence that I would make them all come true. They were bestsellers in the bookstore in my mind! I bought into them all. Charles Dickens would have been proud of my own version of Great Expectations.

Along my journey, I was also prone to rewrite and alter such stories, even write associated stories linked to them.

But none ever were or came true because all turned out to be fantasy stories. They were all in my head and designed to alter my self-perception.

Don't get me wrong, it's great to have positive dreams; but when your happiness hinges on such stories coming true, you can write the perfect plot with pain as your central character. The hope or expectations born of such stories means you are not fully present and letting your life unfold as intended. You do this in a place of fear.

When the story you've written doesn't come true, you will have opened the door for suffering to fill the pages of your life. Regret and guilt may express themselves fluently as you struggle and refuse to accept that you might have been wrong.

The best example of this is in romantic relationships. When we meet someone that excites us, we start to plan. We want to plan, then replan the plan. It's plan mania! This is it, we declare, the real love of my life is here! We plan the wedding, the kids, and assume this person is our soul mate or twin flame. This is your mind's way of securing a safe and secure future for you.

Unfortunately, your mind is not the source of love – it just thinks it is – and when you try and take control of love and set a new agenda other than what the universe has planned for you, you simply invite disappointment and unnatural outcomes into your life.

What if your relationship indeed has deep purpose, but is not intended to last for the rest of your life?

What if someone *even more* suited to you will grace your life in the future?

The significant relationships you are wanting will not generally arise when you seek them, because the ones you were intended to have will always unfold when you are not looking. They will enter when you and the other person are energetically ready. Not when the calendar entry you made has been reached. Seeking and setting deadlines is mired in the energy of need.

The most productive stories to tell yourself are about your past, for they are done. You might even get the telling of them right if your mind has not been distorted by painful memories and bitter emotions.

We all need to be aware that pain can be the editor that exaggerates any negatives in our stories, and that we are all guilty of rewriting history, so it serves to protect and promote our sometimes-distorted egos!

As you become more aware, you will come to understand that you are likely to experience pain by simply living, and that is normal. Hope will not dispel it. It's how you deal with that pain that matters.

My father always used to say to me, "It's only pain, it won't kill you." How wise he turned out to be.

You can process pain, witness the learnings it has for you and become the author of a wonderful self-help manuscript that changes your life for the better. Alternatively, you can go into the five stages of grief, and write stories of horror and despair that you may never get over or feel the need to spend lots of energy suppressing.

I know what I'd prefer!

People have often said that they feel sorry for me, because I've had some difficult experiences. I am grateful for their care but now know better than to buy-into such naïve views.

Firstly, many people have had far worse experiences than me.

Secondly, the more challenges and pain we have in life, the more opportunities we have to expand and grow beyond our illusions of self. So, I consider the life and pain I have had to be a privilege of sorts! Without the shadow of any doubt, it has enhanced my self-awareness, and opened the door to many new and wonderful possibilities, including writing this and other books.

It's the people who don't take the chances they're given to learn that I feel compassion for. They may keep themselves safe, but they limit their opportunities for expansion.

When you run at fire, rather than away from it, you might get burned, but you might also save things that are precious to you – like your integrity.

The events that take place in your life are orchestrated through you, to help you expand and reveal more and more about your true self. The way I look at them is that they arise from the will of God. They are of love and will not harm the truth of you. What they can do, if you embrace them, is to bring you closer to what truly is.

Collective Stories

For centuries, humanity has used stories to pass information down through the generations and support their cultures. Many of these are of great value and interest to those hearing or telling them.

However, such stories are also likely to enunciate the beliefs and biases that were held by the conditioned minds that told them. History is normally written by those in charge and those who won – the ruling class, in tandem with any media or academics they employ. Accordingly, much of it is distorted to suit the author.

The pain of the past is thus a major issue that humanity has yet to come to terms with – there is so much resentment held between individuals, societies, and nations because of the ego-centric stories told by past collectives.

If we all understood the power of letting-go pain, we would have a far happier world.

Humanity has also long held the common collective belief that it has the intelligence to predict the future. Open the newspaper, or turn on the evening news, and you are bound to find reports by so-called experts telling audiences what they can expect. Often their predictions are based on the originator's own preconditioned hopes and self-interested needs. In all likelihood, people believe them because they too believe that IQ is the proud owner of an all-knowing crystal ball.

The reality is that the world does not work this way, because of how we co-create with divine forces through choice. Our minds only have so much power and control.

The Magic of the Is-ness

We can never be fully present and in-love with our lives as they are, unless we are present in our Is-ness. In other words, accepting of what IS.

Anything else is a fallacy or fictional story of the unaccepting mind. Not accepting where you are in life can keep you trapped in a fairy tale of illusions, or a dungeon of despair.

Lingering pain and confusion is a great indicator that you have become stuck in such an illusion of the mind. Illusion and confusion are best friends after all!

But if you listen to your heart, it will have you learning, healing, and moving on to the next chapter in your life. When you start to venture into the realms of higher conscious awareness and the way our lives really unfold, you can begin to embrace concepts of co-creation and acceptance, free yourself of the needs of the mind, and can more intuitively allow the universe to assist you in creating the life you want or desire. A new start may beckon.

Sometimes you *will* get what you need in life, but only temporarily; for the universe will eventually challenge it for you, to expose any validations that remain, so you can reassess them and change.

Only when you need nothing, will you get everything in perpetuity. Love is no thing and ultimately the source of everything. That's the dichotomy of the earthly experience in which we have chosen to partake.

Applying the Arc can bring you more fully into a state of being present and, once you find your own energy of presence, you will be able to simply drop into it at will, no matter where you are. Since everything can only ever happen in the now moment, presence is also critical if you want to manifest a particular outcome and new possibilities. You cannot be anywhere but present when you are connected to your source self, or soul.

Magical relationships can also arise when you are in presence, for the other person can connect to you on a deeper level. Because you are in your purity, you can feel and express your truth freely and have it interacted with, by theirs.

When the other person does the same with you, infinite possibilities exist for love to be present between all involved. Love has the infinite power to create and enhance relationships between people if we allow it to do so.

The infinity symbol is a visual representation of this infinite possibility. It is how all loving beings communicate in the universe.

It works like this:

- I feel, I express.
- You listen and receive, then feel and express.
- This can go on in perpetuity.

This continuous feedback loop in turn provides the basis for truth and love to be present, creating many new and joyful stories between different souls.

Such stories can also promote learning. It's less common than learning from pain simply because, when pain comes, we often want to get out of its clutches as soon as we can. When our circumstances are joyous, we feel less inclined to learn and change, we just enjoy what is even though the joy brings us more easily into presence.

Imagine a world where we all actively learned in the energy of joy, during the good times, not just the bad!

Of course, even bad experiences can become joyous when we love the learnings that arise, more than the pain that we feel. As we master the art of allowing pain to pass through us quickly, we can value periods of discomfort, which can be become increasingly short-lived.

The more you master the Arc, the less impact unpleasant experiences will have on the stories you tell yourself, because you will have the wisdom to know that all is happening for a reason. You will become more resilient and emotionally potent. Once you have become aligned with it consistently, it will give you a sense of being composed and centred, which will then be reflected in the stories you create, particularly the stories about yourself.

Knowing how life truly works can bring you greater peace and solitude, as you become more accepting of all that unfolds. We do not need to die to rest in peace – that story is a falsehood! By applying the Arc, we can effectively erect our own tombstone for the worried person we once were and celebrate our own rebirth into a new experience of wonder. We can be at peace with our lives and all that has unfolded, even if sometimes it felt like going through hell to get there. This can create our own form of resurrection.

I now look back at all the uncomfortable experiences in my life through a lens of gratitude. I am much more at peace, not because I have been able to alter what happened, but because I have learnt so much from them, and arisen to a new place of self-awareness.

Self-acceptance is an important aspect of accepting the Is-ness of life. Accepting and forgiving yourself is a great priority along your path.

I have certainly found self-forgiveness and self-acceptance to be a great challenge, given the perfectionistic traits I developed early in my life. I suspect I am not alone! I have always found it easier to forgive others than to forgive myself. This has made finding peace in my own presence to be a great challenge until now!

Patience Becomes a Strength

Once we have imagined a story for our lives, our minds often become inherently impatient to realise that story and want to move at a speed beyond that of nature. But that is a waste of energy – have you ever tried speeding up the waves of the ocean, or the erosion of sand on the beach?

Instead, we must trust that the right events will enter our lives when they are meant to; thus the application of the Arc will require you to slow down, tune into your truth, trust that the universe has your best interests at heart, and be in the energy of patience.

As you come into alignment with this, you will tread with greater surety through the chapters of your story. It may not feel this way initially but, by slowing down your steps, you will become more certain and solid, making miss-steps far less likely.

I certainly needed to learn this the hard way. Impatience was never my strength, because I was obsessed with external achievements, until I discovered that it only caused me pain, because it was birthed out of the belief that I knew better than the universe about how my path was meant to unfold. And I valued external outcomes more than I valued my own internal happiness for many years.

Aligning with your true path requires you to understand that your inner reality will *eventually* translate into an outer reality more in line with your heart's desires, though not necessarily at the speed you want.

Once you accept this, far less effort will be required to take great leaps forward and, ultimately, the more you learn to slow down, the more you can't help but speed up!

An Illuminating Personal Example

I was fortunate enough once to meet a very beautiful woman with whom I felt an immediate deep soul connection. We briefly became casual friends, but one day I could not resist asking her out. I really wanted to explore the intense connection I felt with her when I looked into her eyes. It was beyond any I had ever felt, to that point in my life.

To my great disappointment she said 'no', then chose to avoid me from that day onward. She had a partner, so I respected her choice and admired the fact that she honoured her partner so intensely. I probably came across as needy, because of the intensity of my feelings. They led me to express unattractive energies and, the truth is, I later realised that I was needy of her attention.

I have faced this truth within me, and now accept that that was the best I could be at that stage of my evolution, particularly in the face of feelings that were so new to me.

This did not stop me going into deep pain. I told lots of stories to myself over the next year about how I wasn't good enough for her, or that she was unfair on me. There were countless stories of woe. Eventually, I found peace in the situation, but only after I realised that I had caused my own pain by writing fictions in the library of my brain about her, and by not stopping to face and release the physical pain of rejection that I felt.

I also had several experiences arise with this woman in my karmic clearing practices. It turned out that she and I had shared multiple past lives together. This explained the intensity of the resonance that I felt towards her. She is a significant soul mate.

I will be forever grateful for the rejection I received from this impressive woman, as ridiculous as this may sound, for it allowed me to grow in many wonderful ways. I faced my demons by using the principles in this book. I certainly learned self-forgiveness. And I came to see her original rejection as a valid choice she was entitled to make, after all it is her life.

Next time, I will know to face any emotions I feel in the moment, rather than allowing myself to go into the blame and shame game, then stay mired in the pain of rejection for an extended period.

Ultimately, my pain lingered, as did my suffering, for much longer than it needed to because I did not deem myself worthy, so I allowed myself to play the role of both victim and martyr. But this was all a choice I made, and I now own it. She did nothing wrong. I was the enemy of my own happiness.

I am now grateful for the experience, as it has assisted with my self-esteem, rather than diminished it. The pain helped me to discover greater truths, which my soul wanted me to know, and in turn I took further steps towards the light within my heart.

What stories are you telling yourself that are built on fantasy. Assumptions and expectations built on false hope, will only ever take you on a journey into disappointment and pain.

Perhaps it's time you changed the source of the author writing your current stories, so you can tune into new plots with inspiring possibilities?

Your heart has its own quill and stands ready to write a light and beautiful autobiography that you can enjoy!

CHAPTER 17

The Love You Truly Seek

Being Pure Love

When we apply the Arc, or other valuable modalities, to assist our awareness journeys, it is important to understand that: you are already what you seek.

Inside you sits your holy grail, awaiting discovery by the only explorer that can find it – YOU. Your heart has the same power as Sir Galahad's heart.

Allowing Self-Love to Overwhelm You

There is much written about finding self-love within you, but your true self already loves you.

It's only the conditioned mind that thinks and tries to convince us that we are not lovable, and tampers with our feelings. With this core and complex wound in our fields and subconscious minds, many of us go through our lives trying to convince those around us that we are valuable and interesting. Image management is just as rife as pain management.

Your belief that you are not enough is usually stopping you from finding the source of true love within you, making you spend enormous levels of energy trying to create a lovable image to others. It's a big mind game, because self-love can never be thought. It must be felt.

Many people convince themselves that they unconditionally love themselves, but this is normally just a thought, no more, because they are thinking it in a strong ego-centric mind that likes to be right. Their truth will surface, however, when their 'tide' goes out.

I know I lived it!

Self-love can only ever be felt in your heart, through the natural connection that love allows. The Arc can help you to remember this through the feelings in your body.

You need to remember that your true self loves you beyond your wildest dreams, and always will. It vibrates in line with the energy of universal love, as it has been since its creation, and as it will forever more. It is the one source of love that you will always be able to rely upon in this life. Others may come and go to assist your journey home, but you heart is your unconditional lover once you uncover it.

In addition, your ego can never be fully satisfied but your heart accepts you no matter what you do. Living as conscious awareness can bring your self-love forth and dismantle your egoic needs for ever increasing levels of safety and externally defined versions of success.

You can either wait until you die to become conscious of this again, or you can become conscious of it now, while you are creating your own heaven in your own life. You are life living a physical life, and the life force within your true self is waiting to show you a divine experience. It wants to live you, not have your mind think that it can live it. It gives you endless experiences to help you work this out.

The consciousness path is calling on you gently to allow this to be possible now! All you need to do is get your thoughts out of the way of the vibration of love within you, and let your soul take you to this forgotten place of deep true love that is unmistakable.

When I feel disappointed that I have not done as well as I could have at anything, I simply go deep within myself to feel the serenity and energy in my heart. This tells me that I am deeply loved and supported, regardless of the circumstances. Any concept of failure melts away in the cauldron of my own love, although if pain arises and offers me the opportunity for higher self-awareness, I will always embrace that gift.

Humanity has dismissed so many natural concepts about our truth, that we have largely lost our way. But now many are waking up in the face of unbearable pain to what is possible in the energy of love.

Finding True Love

We love to be in love, and constantly talk of finding true love. However, the quest for true love is widely misrepresented.

The first misrepresentation is that true love can only ever be found with a romantic partner. This is not true – it can be established with any other human being, and we need to broaden our thinking in this way.

Another misrepresentation is that anyone can find true love. But true love can only ever be established when two people, who both know their own truths, come together in a blended experience together.

Unless you are highly conscious, therefore, you will never find true love, because you will need love too much, to fill the metaphorical hole in your heart. It doesn't matter how good looking, intelligent or talented your intended partner is – unless you are the energy of true love, the universe cannot and will not bestow true love upon you.

This is where the Arc can help, for love is a vibrational match – always – and souls recognise each other through vibration. In this respect, love is quite scientific.

As discussed above, our vibration in this life is defined by the rate at which our body cells and energy fields oscillate and vibrate. When we enter this life, we bring an essence with us, represented in our energy fields. This essence has the energies we need to fulfil our stated life path, but also contains negative energies that we can delete or modify to enhance our energetic experiences. Our essence can also carry energies borrowed from other beings to assist us with our mission on Earth. This essence generates our vibration, and the clearer the essence, the higher our vibration.

Once you have attained your full connection with your own self, you can then potentially make a vibrational match with another person who lives in their own light like you. True love can then enter your life for real.

We won't find true love by chasing love and trying to control or own it. We must let it own and become us. It will enter our life when the infinite intelligence of the universe knows that two souls are ready to experience this incredible and unbreakable bond of pure love.

Just about every couple I talk to that seems remotely happy tells me that they think they are experiencing true or pure love. Frankly, the majority are not, for they do not know what true love feels like.

They are no-doubt experiencing love. However, love has different levels of purity, and this is determined by the needs and fears inherent in the belief structures we take into a relationship.

In the nine romantic relationships I have had in my life, each time I thought I had found true love. I know now that I had not, for in each experience I was still carrying unhelpful conditioning. These relationships were based on love, but not absolutely pure love.

It doesn't mean we should exit a relationship that is not true love. All relationships ultimately serve both partners to expand, and in doing so get closer to connecting to their own source of self-love – their hearts. Two partners on a journey to consciousness can advance their relationship to true love together. I have witnessed this.

A soul experiencing true love has no need for the other soul to love it whatsoever. True love is devoid of need, yet full of desire. A person in the energy of true love does not judge because they fully accept the other. And all this is felt, not thought. In a state of true love, thinking about love is unnecessary because we already are it. We don't need to believe in it for we have gone beyond beliefs to the state of knowing.

Ask yourself honestly, have you ever felt this kind of love? Do not think the answer, let your guts tell you. I've not felt it with another person yet, only within myself and with angelic beings, who taught me how to merge my energy fields with theirs.

If you haven't felt true love, don't give up! Just do the work to find your own true love first. If you have a current partner, they can always hold your hand and journey down this path with you. This is called conscious relating.

Of course, you may not want to pursue true love because the path to arrive at this advanced state takes great courage to traverse. You must try to be love, rather than fall into it, so that you have love to share with someone at the same point of evolution.

The Arc can help you discover this much-coveted gift of true love.

Tinder, I suspect, cannot!

The Soul Mate Mythology

Western cultures often refer to the wonder of finding a soul mate in life. The soul mate concept is unfortunately misunderstood as well.

The truth is that we have many soul mates that accompany us through eternity, lifetime after lifetime. They can play different roles in each incarnation.

I know, for example, that my mother in this life was married to me in a past life. She is a soul mate.

All souls are connected, so in a sense we are all soul mates. However, soul families share experiences together over many centuries and even eons, and help each other to gain the lessons we need to receive.

When we meet a soul with whom we have had a past connection, we will often feel this connection in our hearts. It can be a powerful love because our souls are remembering each other deeply. There may also be energetic karma that they may need to dissolve, and this can be the purpose of the chance meeting between them.

If a romantic connection feels very strong and loving, there is a good chance that the other person is a soul mate.

A soul mate is different, however, to a twin flame. Soul mates come and go as we journey through life. They unite with us as needed, then exit once their role is complete in this life. On the other hand, although a twin flame also travels with us through eternity, we have only one twin flame in the universe, and that person is the opposite side of our soul.

This aligns with the concept of yin and yang. Our relationship with our twin flame is unbreakable throughout our eternal thread. There is a deep trust between twin flames because their souls both recognise that they are truly one.

When both sides are vibrationally ready for a powerful and true love, their meeting is dynamic. Imagine two souls in their full light and truth, coming together to share a passionate and romantic exchange. This type of reunion is possible and will be periodically experienced as their respective threads unfold. Since twin flames are the opposite sides of the same complete soul, they can experience a blending of energies that is extraordinary, and this effectively allows both souls to feel a sense of being complete when they are together. However, the relationship can also be testing if neither are yet to find their full light. Two souls that are the mirror image of each other, yet add together to form one complete soul, is a difficult concept to grasp.

There are many articles about twin flame experiences on the internet for those who wish to explore this phenomenon in greater detail or suspect that they may have experienced these circumstances in their own lives. Famous twins throughout history include Jesus and Mary Magdalene, and from Ancient Egyptian fame King Osiris and Isis.

There are many others, and one day you will have your own twin flame reunion if you choose to; though it may be extremely testing, and such experiences are believed to be only bestowed on those who are ready to face the intense spiritual challenges that it brings forth. It can be more of a spiritual learning opportunity rather than a romantic fairy tale in some incarnations.

All relationships are essentially experiments to help us grow because they hold up a mirror to our insecurities so we can face them, but the twin flame version is regarded as next level in its intensity. Indeed, the energy between two twin flames can be very powerful and all-consuming, because it is bringing forth the possibility of unconditional love with another.

Although this incredible blending of love is not fully available until both partners are in their own space of pure self-love, our souls do want us to experience at some point in our evolution because it is so wonderful. It may be initially resisted by our minds, as the experience can serve to bring forth very deep conditioning for clearing. This can be emotionally painful, and many twins will flee a twin flame experience once it begins, because it is often so challenging and intense to endure; unlike a soul mate experience, which can be far more serene and peaceful.

I have had one incredibly intense experience in my life with a woman who I suspect MAY have been my twin flame. When I was near her, I felt an intense soul connection, and just being in her presence created intense waves of physical vibration throughout my chakra system. Her presence seemed to connect me straight to my own heart and hers. I know from the past life work I have done that she and I are, at the very least, soul mates; but whether it was ever any more than that I may never know.

The way I felt about her fitted every experience I have ever read about twin flames. However, as she was in a relationship with another person, I never got to explore this situation with any depth in the physical realm.

The Arc can help you find your own way to a twin flame experience should you wish it. If you want to meet your ultimate partner, the fastest way to that experience is to devote energy to your own evolution, not to go online. The higher your vibration becomes; the higher will be the vibrational match that you establish with another.

You need to do the work on you to experience a love that's true.

CHAPTER 18

You Will Not Be Alone

Sharing Your Journey Inward

Tuning in or meditating on a feeling is normally best done on your own; thus the path to knowing yourself requires you to be alone and go inward often, until you are self-reflecting on a regular basis. Only you can feel your own heart, and ultimately find your way 'home' and through the front door.

To develop the Arc, I spent a lot of time alone. I seemed to have a lot of conditioning to work through, and I was intent on taking this process to an advanced place.

That does not mean you need to be single to do the same. Whatever your life circumstances, you can still apply the Arc. In fact, if you are in a loving relationship, you may expand faster if you receive conscious support from another. Relationships can help you see yourself in the mirror and will undoubtedly help you see any limiting beliefs you may hold.

Becoming of higher consciousness will almost certainly require you to release pain from your past. This can be confronting for a person close to you, who may witness you processing your pain. It is important that those around you understand that your self-reflection, and perhaps changing moods, is not a reflection on your current circumstances or relationship with them.

The point is that this type of deep personal investigation may worry someone who does not share what you are experiencing, or who does not want to come on the same journey. They may not be open to you expressing the emotions you may need to express, or they may find your changing patterns of behaviour to be unsettling, because they are more accustomed to normal ways of being.

Just like the child who is taught at a young age that only positive emotions are valued in this world, some people will naturally carry that thinking into relationships. All you can do is explain to them openly what you are now allowing to take place in your life and ask them to support you in your quest to be more self-aware. Most likely, they will be the benefactors of the lighter, happier you that will emerge as you become truer to yourself.

I had this experience in a relationship, and it got awkward at times, having to explain why I was experiencing and releasing negative emotions when, on the surface, my life was in a good place. I had to explain to my partner that I was releasing decades-old pain. However, she was not overly receptive to my path, and was concerned that my emotions related to her. This put undue pressure on our relationship.

By the same token, I have viewed some advanced relationships where both partners support the other on their personal journey and provide a 'cheer squad' to help lift their partners to higher consciousness.

You are Never on Your Own

There may also be times when going inward may be better served by being alone.

I have found that when I am processing a significant energy or pain from my past, I sometimes need to seek solitude.

If you do the same, you may feel alone in those times, at least in the physical world.

But the important thing to realise is that you are never actually on your own. Your soul and your guides are always with you, even if you can't see, hear, or touch them. They will never leave your side. Your soul is the eternal you and it will love you on your journey to enlightenment forever.

The deeper my relationship with myself has become, the less I need contact with other people. Need is the appropriate word here.

The fact is, as you lighten up and become more of the real-you, you start to find your true tribe of people – those who share your interests and value you fully for who and what you are. You are more likely to discontinue relationships with people who do not value you. This can be temporarily disruptive. However, it can also transform your life for the better.

Under Newton's third law, every action on earth has an equal and opposite reaction. Therefore, when you change the energy that you put out, it changes the energy coming back at you.

Self-Acceptance on the Path?

As I have journeyed through the Arc and interacted with metaphysical energies, I have gone through periods of worrying that I will not be readily accepted by others, and may even be persecuted for my advanced understandings and practices.

You may also experience this self-imposed fear as you step more and more into the metaphysical aspects of yourself.

For periods, I even went into a kind of withdrawal energy, when I was exploring many of these new concepts, because I struggled to talk openly about many of the abnormal happenings taking place for me.

I never wanted to stop my processes and learnings, but I felt threatened by the potential for judgement by others who had not had the same experiences. I unnecessarily separated myself at times and underestimated the curiosity of others.

Many people will be interested in your journey as you adopt more advanced ways of living. Of course some may also be critical. For the sake of those who remain mired in normality, you may at first need to limit what you disclose when around them, for they are not ready to hold the concepts you want to share and may criticise you to protect their own status. You can become more authentic when you find that new tribe.

I have become more committed to authenticity as I have advanced through the Arc, and this has opened the doorway for me to meet people who are on a similar path to greater self-awareness. I haven't had to arrange this. People have entered my life through synchronicity, as and when I needed them, or they needed me.

It's important to see every interaction with another human being as a chance to learn more about yourself. We choose every experience we are exposed to. As a result, every event or interaction is a mirror into ourselves, if we have the foresight and insight to witness it from this perspective. Remember you are here on Earth to open to the truth of yourself and to experience what you, as the real you, are capable of experiencing!

Ultimately, the Arc will give you greater connection to yourself and to the rest of the world. But initially you may prefer to seek greater solitude as you work through your buried pain.

Eventually, as you discover what and who you really are, you will feel more inclined to be the true-you, no matter what you do and no matter who else is watching you.

THE POSSIBILITIES AWAITING YOU

CHAPTER 19

Manifesting Beyond the Mind

Different Sources of Manifestation

Manifestation is a well-known concept, and many spiritual and religious books are well versed on the subject. Manifestation basically refers to something becoming real after initially being a mere dream, concept or thought.

The entire 3D world in which we live has in fact been created from manifestation. To become real, everything we see around us in our 3D feedback loop was once a dream, concept or thought. The combination of energy, in the form of a concept or image, and effort, in the form of doing, creates reality. One might say that the merging of metaphysical consciousness and physical effort lead to things coming true. A conscious thought or dream does not exist until we do the work in the material world to bring it into our dimensional reality.

There are different sources of manifestation. We can manifest from our minds through thoughts, or from our hearts through dreams. Both can lead to the creation of physical things if they are supported by human effort.

Most human beings live predominantly in their minds; even people on the spiritual path tend to, because they only access the soul in the process of intermittent meditation. Accordingly, many things in this world are born out of thoughts from the human mind, and quite often from the conditioned ego. This is not bad – it just is. It is the logical outcome of the way we have existed for centuries.

Unfortunately, however, our world has many structures and manifested outcomes we may not find appealing. This is because they may have been derived or manifested out of ego, not love. War, and the industrial military complex that supports it, are the worst examples of fear or ego-based manifestations. There are countless others, as detailed further in my book *Where Your Happiness Hides*.

If more things were manifested from the energy of love, instead of the fear, can you imagine what our lives, and our world, would be like? As our world moves into the higher vibrations that are currently evolving for us, this will come; it will just take time!

As an individual, however, applying the principles in this book and specifically the Arc, you can manifest more from a place of love in your own life. You do not need to wait for the person next to you to do it first, or for the rest of the world! In fact, you can change your life for the better quite quickly, once you master manifesting from the desires of your own heart. This loving state will then ripple out into the world as others witness your renaissance or rebirth. It will be like throwing a rock into a pond and watching the waves unfold.

Manifesting the life that you want is a wonderful destination that the power of the Arc can give you, when it is applied out of the purity of your heart, your centre point. It's all about vibrations. Your vibration is everything on this journey.

Given that everything we witness in this world is light, everything has its own vibration.

While love operates at high vibrations, bad and dense things are represented by low vibrational light waves. People often speak of darkness in their lives, but there is truly no such thing. All is light. Even space is full of light, acting as a conduit for the light of the sun and other energies; we just can't generally see the light until it strikes low vibrational objects, slows down and lights it up.

Manifesting with the ego is therefore much more likely to result in creating things at lower vibrations, than creating things with the higher vibration of love. When you apply the principles in this book with integrity and regularity, you can't help but get closer and closer to the vibration of love that-you-already-are, manifesting a life that will make you happier and more evolved.

Clearing your limiting beliefs, and allowing conscious receptivity and application to enter your own universe, will take you closer to the vibration you were born to be. Once applied, this will give you the power to manifest the life and circumstances of your dreams.

How Do I Manifest Out of Love?

The love within you has the power to bring inspiration to your mind and embed it in your imagination; thus manifesting from your heart commences with feelings, then initiates a dream that will lead the mind to start formulating new possibilities. Once you receive these imaginings, you then step in and do the doing to make your dream come true. Like everything, this process combines the physical and metaphysical.

Of course, the higher your vibration the higher the possibility of manifesting from your heart. Once you enter your light, you become the alchemist, the full creator.

Here is the process, which I have received directly from metaphysical guidance:

- Feel the energy of your dream in your body,
- Visualise it as best you can and feel your love for it,
- Go into the state of awareness you use to create your connection to your true self, such as meditation. Your mind can assist, but only as a facilitator,
- Imagine you placing your dream in the 'fire' that burns inside

your heart or chest (like the imagery often found in Christian churches of Jesus Christ),
- Place around that 'fire' any obstacles that might stand in the way of this manifestation,
- Ask your heart to then explode its loving energy outwards, to destroy the barriers to creation, and send your dream to the universe to enact co-creation,
- Be ready to step into your dream and any synchronicity that arises, for you and through you, knowing that the universe will support you to the extent that your dream aligns with love, and
- Apply your physical and mental capabilities alongside love to bring your dream into reality. Resistance is not an option if you want fulfilment of your dream

All in this world is energy before it is manifested into physicality. As energies coalesce, nothing can become something.

Remember that the time frames set by your mind for a dream to manifest may not align with the potential for universal energies to coalesce. So be patient. Let it come and step in at the right time.

The further into the Arc you go the more likely you are to master this art.

Combining Love with Logic

The most potent combination from which to create anything wonderful, is to allow the heart to dream. The heart then gives an idea to the mind, to organise what is needed to be done in a logical and efficient manner. This is where the mind excels. It is good at organising and planning what needs to be done, to ground or earth the dream into our 3D reality.

The body is the doer. Its physical capabilities allow concepts to be built into reality.

This natural coordination of our whole selves is how we create divine outcomes. Manifestation is possible because of our inherent state of duality.

Manifesting in Tension

A common spiritual saying is that our intentions determine where we place our attention. This determines what we do and achieve in life.

Easy to say, but how does the power of intention work, and how does it align with the concept of co-creation?

When we create an intention, our minds communicate to our souls what we want. This, in turn, is then communicated to the universe through the soul's unbreakable connection with the universal field. Of course, our egos may work against these intentions if we lack the necessary alignment between heart, body, and mind. Accordingly, we may unknowingly sabotage the manifestation of what we want. We may instead manifest what we need out of fear-based thinking.

Assuming the necessary alignment is in place, however, we then go into a place of tension with universal forces. Through synchronicity and other supportive processes, the universe can and will bring us the necessary opportunities to which we need to apply our energies.

This doesn't mean sitting back and waiting for divine intervention to do it all for you. When you step into what is possible, like I outlined in my explanation of the Arc, this sends a clear message to the universe within you, that you are ready to co-create what you are imagining. You are the creator, ready to create with love and then physical effort. From the birth of a new idea, new beginnings can take shape.

Many dreamers, normally thought leaders or inventors, need doers to create a more wonderful world. The same applies to the life you lead! You can be both the dreamer and the doer.

Why not allow your inner reality to manifest an outer reality that you will love? This is the conscious individual's superpower. You can manifest what you need or manifest what you truly want. Tuning into your own heart can show you what it truly desires for you. Abundance awaits – don't keep it waiting!

CHAPTER 20

What Becomes Possible

The Lost Art of Being a Human Light Being

Scientists are constantly trying to analyse and understand the Earth and the universe around us, even though a full understanding is beyond the capabilities of our human intelligence. Ironically, we spend relatively little time and effort trying to understand ourselves. This situation gives us lots of information but limits us significantly.

We are also prone to distract ourselves from our inner pain and potential self-understandings through engaging with external stimuli, like the internet and television shows. Here we invest our life force in observing the lives of others, rather than our own. Technology has become a huge part of our lives and is therefore important, but when we spend more time looking at our cell phones than into our own hearts, they truly are well named.

When we focus on things that are removed from ourselves, we live a lesser existence than we are capable of, individually and collectively.

Here are the differing states we can all generally chose to live within:

- **Totally in the mind, or ego** – in this state, you exist solely at the direction of your egocentric mind. It makes the choices for you: where you live, what you do, who you love, what you don't like and so on. It is all founded in thinking. This thinking may be conditioned, however, and is therefore influenced by your past in different ways, as well as any enduring pain that you are experiencing. In this state, you are in your individual state of personality, known as separation consciousness; and you may not trust your intuition, or even hear it, because you are separated from your true self.

- **In the mind, with occasional interactions with your feelings** – in this state you live primarily in the mind, but you give some credibility to your feelings in making your choices in life. You have evolved beyond just thought. You have fleeting engagements with your soul. You know how to access your intuition to some degree. But your awareness of the truth of yourself and thus your consciousness is low, and you remain in a state of separation consciousness.

- **In the mind, but you understand the power of self-awareness** – this is typical of many spiritually aware people. They know they are more than a mind, and they consciously try to access their soul, and the powers beyond, through intermittent meditation practices and other mindfulness practices. You have awakened, and you are intent on becoming purer of heart. You are conscious and can go further if you choose. You may have attended self-help courses, watched podcasts and read books that are full of great theory. But, because those teaching you are most likely in the same paradigm, you may not be truly aware of what is possible for a conscious human being and how far you can take this. You can only choose from the options presented, and only those you can understand.

In this state, you are most likely in your individualised personality most of the time; but you are aware of the concept of unity consciousness, and in meditation you venture into it temporarily. You are moving closer to higher consciousness awareness.

- **You become the soul all the time** – this is an advanced state of consciousness and is akin to being in a constant state of meditation. In this place, you are in constant connection with the soul, and with the physical realms at the same time, all the time. You are in duality 24/7. Your in-built adviser is constantly letting you know how you could choose to live your life in alignment with purity.

You are either naturally born with a high vibration, or you have done the work to substantially clear the 'pipe' between your mind and your soul. You are truly whole. Your soul knows that you are in a high enough place of purity to allow it to become the core driver of your mind and body. You are entering a phase of great advancement and transformation. Personal alchemy can take place in this state, as your soul takes over the living of your life, including the way you think and the way your body heals. The soul will determine this through its access to infinite wisdom and higher vibrational energies.

The soul has incredible capabilities beyond anything most of us can imagine. Consider the fact that your soul is eternal (i.e. does not age), has access to all your current and 'past 'memories, can relinquish all your karma, is omnipresent (i.e. can consciously be in multiple places and dimensions at once), and can communicate with every other being in the universe at will. What do you think might be possible for a human that becomes more and more aligned with this energy?

In this energy, your divine path can unfold as you arise from the ashes of your past like the legendary Phoenix. You are consciousness living a human existence, in a greater state of happiness, and you have powers way beyond any you ever imagined. Your light being is able to merge and integrate with your human being.

> In this state, you become your universal self. You are in unity consciousness.
>
> I repeat: the merger with your full light being only occurs once you are in the vibration of love. But your soul will burst forth when you are ready for that.

Unfortunately, this last state of being is one that was lost to most in humanity thousands of years ago. Jesus and other holy beings have attempted to remind us of our possibilities but, for the most part, the extent of what is possible as a human being living on the Earth has become lost in the annals of time, conditioning, and human thinking. We have become shadows of what we really are, because the radiant lights within us have ceased to be allowed to cast their beams onto our lives.

We think that modern man is more advanced than our ancient predecessors, but this is far from the case, for many in ancient times understood these principles. They worked with nature around them and the metaphysical realms to manifest.

Religions as a rule do not comprehend this possibility, for they too were largely constructed through the power of the human mind. So don't expect to hear these truths in church on a Sunday morning!

I have experienced all four of these states of being, so I can speak with my truth about each of them. My experience with the last one is still unfolding into my light under the guidance of my mentors, but is well advanced, and I know it will continue to evolve until I die.

Many spiritual books and circles refer to what is possible when we fully connect to our dual nature in this most evolved state as 'As Above, So Below'.

In terms of the Arc, this relates to the latter phases, like Phases 8 and 9, when we have the consciousness possible in the spirit realm (which we all have after we die and consciously return to the metaphysical) yet are very much alive in our current incarnation and can apply that consciousness to our physical life on Earth.

Achieving this state of being of 'As Above, So Below' is extremely rare, and has historically applied to only a minuscule number of people in recent millennia. Arriving in this energy can be described as coming HOME to the truth of what you really are.

The energetic forces or vibrations now radiating onto the Earth are, however, very supportive of the advancement into this high state of evolution. It is, however, a matter of awareness and choice. The universe is ready to support all of us on this journey, should we choose to take it. This is not a small decision, for it will put you at odds with many of society's normal ways of thinking and take commitment to self.

Great Mysteries Can Arise from Within You

When you reach a stage of complete connection with your soul, you can connect to infinite intelligence and be always in your light. In this state, you are lighter by definition and therefore experience greater happiness and bliss. However, you may also develop new psychic/metaphysical abilities and wisdom that you didn't know you had. In essence, love is connecting you to higher vibrations and energies that exist beyond mankind's normal perceptions.

It's a bit like having your own private Google system that can give you access to infinite intelligences, as are relevant to your circumstances. You just type in your enquiries and the light communicates to you with the answers that you need to know.

These new advanced abilities could include:

- telepathy,
- astral travel capabilities and the ability to remember where your consciousness travels to, for instance as you sleep,
- omnipresence, or the ability to be present through your consciousness in multiple places at once,

- the ability to communicate with beings beyond this dimension through sight, sound or feeling,
- being able to connect to the souls of others and communicate at that level at any time,
- being able to sense into another's chakra systems and feel into their energies to assist them,
- the ability to sense into the likely future or the past by accessing into the Akashic Records,
- the ability to heal your own illnesses,
- to have the universe channel wisdom through your body, in spoken word and written form – this is called channelling,
- the ability to throw sexual energy at another person from a distance, or during tantric sex,
- the capability to remember your dreams with greater clarity and to change the energy inherent within them for many of them constitute memories,
- the capability to merge your energy field with another's field, to create a blended field and to enhance the love between you,
- being able to witness the white light of all things, through the third eye, and
- the ability to blend your field and energies with the whole of the universal field,

I have personally experienced each of these as I have applied the Arc. There is no doubt that many other capabilities are possible, as we are all unique; my own experiences continue to evolve every day of my life.

I am grateful that I have been gifted with these experiences, but I never take them for granted, nor do I believe they are an achievement of any kind. They occur when my soul wants them to. I cannot demand that they take place, and if I misuse my gifts or use them out of ego only, they can be taken away as quickly as they arrive by my soul.

I have had occasions where people I meet have told me that they feel like I look through them and into their deeper knowing. This is true to some degree because I can connect intentionally to their soul if their soul allows it. Mind-to-mind connection is far less efficient. People with high EQ tend to do aspects of this naturally. However, it can be far deeper and intentional once your vibration rises.

Unless you are aware of the possibility of activating deeper aspects of yourself, you will not be able to make the choice to do so. And, of course, you may not then choose it anyway. That is okay – it is your life and nobody else owns your life!

But if you were to choose to do these things, then you probably could, for we are all equal.

So, yes, you could become psychic, though it would not be your mind psychically connecting with others, it would be your soul. Your soul is the source of all psychic experiences, so it would determine when and how you have them, if you are vibrationally ready to do so. If not, you may need to 'work' on your vibration.

I fell into this second category. My experiences only started after my second divorce and once I started my journey through the Arc.

Soon after I attended a psychic testing day, just for fun. What unfolded was way beyond my expectations. I found out that my soul could read the energy of objects, diagnose the medical history of people I had never met, access the Akashic Records in meditation, and perform telekinesis on light objects. This was a big surprise to me because I had zero expectations in this regard.

My personal experiences with the metaphysical realm have become more common and wonderful as my vibration has risen; but my best experiences rarely occur when I am thinking about them or trying to do them. My soul determines if I am to be graced by such incredible gifts and opportunities. My mind does not.

For those who wish to make the same choices as me, higher vibrations are making it more and more possible to increase your self-awareness, dissolve karma, and address limiting beliefs. This work can help you to bring forth your true self with the will of God. That is the key purpose of this book. To make you aware of what is possible, so you can make whatever choice you feel you should make in your best interests.

Being My Buzz

Since I have mastered the ability to be in my own presence, I call my connection to my soul: my buzz. When I hear and feel this buzz, I know I am fully present with my true self in that moment. I'm sure this experience is different for everyone, but this is what it's like for me.

I feel and hear a buzzing noise in my whole body. Initially I could detect this buzz when I was semi-conscious in bed, because in those moments my mind was substantially shut down. In this place, my 'pipe' was more open, and I was able to recognise the universal energy of my soul.

As I have advanced down my path through the Arc, the sound of my inner energy has become more and more prominent. I now feel it in my form all day long, particularly when I focus on it and drop into my presence with intention. It has become progressively louder and yet finer. I compare it to the sound of a lightbulb buzzing away, although I know that others can't hear it!

What I am hearing is the sound of love or ohm – the universal vibration of love, for at our core that is what we all are. I believe this vibrational pitch within me is gradually rising to align with higher vibrations. Another word for this vibration is resonance.

The possibility for you to hear this is within you too.

If you have ever listened to solfeggios on YouTube, you will understand what I mean. These vibrational pieces are available in different levels of resonance and are designed to help you lift your vibration and self-awareness. Why not give them a try?

When your body and even your mind starts to align with the resonance that you already are, the more your soul will know you are ready for it to gain ascendency over your ego. It is the intelligent force that is allowing your ego to be gradually dissolved and your true vibration of self-love to be felt.

Different Heights of Inspiration

When you reach a state of connection with your universal self, the Arc will help your soul to show you what and who you came here to be and to know. This awareness is likely to overwhelm you and inspire you to new heights.

Before you were born onto this planet in the physical form, you agreed to a divine life plan that you are encoded to fulfil. However, one of our great challenges is to open to the truth in our hearts so that we can feel-into this intended destiny. Few ever find it, for few people know how to find it or that it even exists. This is a core purpose of this book – to show you what is possible.

But those heights will differ greatly for every person, because we all come here with different tests and opportunities, rendering comparisons between us irrelevant and unhelpful. You will never know the full force of your being until you are it!

Until you reach this point of evolution, you can only catch glimpses of it through practices that temporarily minimise the impact of your mind on your conscious awareness, such as meditation or other spiritual modalities.

But as long as you keep taking steps towards the true-you, you will catch these glimpses. All steps taken are valuable. Even applying the principles embodied in the Arc periodically will enhance your sense of self gradually over time, so keep at it!

Many people, particularly those on the spiritual path, speak of finding their life's purpose. The reality is that this can never be thought;

it must be felt. If it's only thought, it is unlikely to be your true divine purpose.

The good news is that we all have a divinity code inside us – in our hearts.

However, the bad news is that it is inactive in most people and will remain so for the rest of their current incarnation, for it will only be activated once an individual is in the light, or in other words has made it home to the truth of themselves in the vibration of love.

A person's divine code is activated by their soul, and it gives that person the choice to be able to make one or a series of divine contributions to the Earth, during their thread on this planet. It is likely to occur once they have overcome their key elements of karma and are close to ascending to higher dimensions. In this energy, they become aware of their divine path and have the support of the universe to enact their divine contribution, for their sake and the sake of others. Perhaps Michelangelo or Albert Einstein found theirs? Only the God within them knows.

The soul knows when an individual is ready for this energetic event. It must be allowed to arise as our conscious awareness rises beyond the limiting vibration of security consciousness. It is sparked by high vibration and unity consciousness. In this, you are in that place of purity.

The Vibration of Universal Love

The path to enlightenment allows the person who reaches their own light to embody the purity of love that they already are. You can be in love or experience love with others, but being the vibration of universal love is next level. Only a relative minority of humans have experienced true unconditional love in recent centuries, because of the density to which we have been subjected.

Universal love is the same as unconditional love. In a state of unconditional love, you have the same power to love like Jesus, or an angel, in that you love everything unconditionally. That means, no matter how the universe responds to you, you will love it with all your heart. This is why Jesus on the cross felt no blame towards those who killed him. He knew the power of universal love coursing through his veins. He did not need to forgive those who harmed him on the cross, because he understood that all happens for purpose. Again, he told me this truth.

You are, of course, already the vibration of universal love. Your conditioned beliefs are just creating a density that stops you feeling-into your full vibration of love, and ultimately experiencing your full light.

We are all connected to the same source of energy and wisdom. You need to remember this and allow it to fully arise within you as your consciousness grows.

The true-you will be ready for a purer form of love with others as a result.

This is a great gift of tuning into your universal self through the Arc.

Compassion Emerges

Imagine a world where enemies resolve their conflicts with compassion for the pain of others. This is a long way from the normal interactions that take place in the energy of righteousness. As a society, do we want to be right or happy? I know which one is more beneficial to love and peace!

When someone reacts badly to something you believe in or say, we always need to realise that they are merely in a place of pain, and not self-love. Compassion is critical when two differing views intersect, and it becomes possible as we become more aware and conscious.

To judge a person for their opinion is not wise or intelligent.

Judgement is always offered on another, out of ignorance for how life truly works. The more aware we become, the more we acknowledge that we are all different people having different experiences in life – we have different families, grow up in different houses, go to different schools and universities, and have different relationships and careers. All of this alters people's conditioned beliefs.

Although our minds often expect alignment, it is therefore extremely naïve to expect complete alignment with anyone, including a romantic partner. We may be similar but can never be completely the same. Compassion emerges as our conscious awareness arises from within us.

Easy Does It!

Contrary to our conditioned thinking, life was meant to be easy. Of course, this can be influenced by the life path you have chosen in this life, and any karma you may have chosen to rebalance. As humans, many of us make life much harder than it needs to be.

Indeed, when you live as the vibration of love – when you are the energy of love, doing what you love and being the source of love – you do not need to try as hard as you probably think you need to do. In fact, in a place of self-love you don't need to try at all. All comes naturally and is largely effortless.

Trying, as a concept, dwells in our egoic minds.

Consider a romantic relationship. Do you think two conscious lovers who deeply love each other equally have to try to make their relationship joyful? Is it hard for them to co-create a great life together? They probably share disagreements and differences, but they intentionally work together to become closer, and even more aligned every time an issue arises. They see disagreements as an opportunity to grow as a couple and individually, not to attribute blame. They understand that the disagreements that arise are just reflective of the different conditioning they possess and can work together to remove. If love is present, the possibilities are endless for their relationship to advance in ever-increasing harmony.

Now picture a couple who are not like this. Their relationship is likely to require hard work and commitment to hold it together. Two egos are likely to be at play and trying to win any conflict that arises. Conflict is probably more common.

As is often said, love what you do and you'll never work another day in your life. In this beautiful place you are supported by synchronicity, as you flow with your destiny and universal support.

You have access to so much more when you become the more-that-you-are. Higher consciousness can take you to this magical place.

I am a very curious person by nature. I couldn't resist the opportunity to apply my inherent curiosity to get to know the most interesting thing in my life: me! When I learned what is possible for human beings, while we are alive, it lit me up, and I have committed to discovering the full extent of the light within me. Who knows where it might take me?

You can choose that totally, or partially too, by following the Arc or similar processes that you prefer. What choice do you want to make?

Don't think it – ask your heart. Feel the decision and remember all choices are valid in the eyes of God, and will not be judged!

CHAPTER 21

Receiving Intelligences

The Inner Whispers I Love

When I first started my journey to higher self-awareness, I found it hard to distinguish between the messages from my mind, my heart, and other beings, like the spirit guides from whom I was receiving intelligences. Over time, it has become much easier to distinguish between them.

The mind can be random and tends to be unsure.

Whereas my heart and messages from guides are clearer, stronger, and do not repeat, unless I ask for them to be repeated. They are always received in perfect timing, just when I need to hear them. You might say the timing is divine; but I can't control them.

The messages from my guides tend to be received from behind my head, between my ears. They are always loving in their intent.

The messages from my soul flood straight into my mind, particularly now that my soul has control of my mind.

One thing that I have had to get used to, but now love, is the fact that I now communicate in multiple directions at once. I may be talking to another human being and being present in that conversation; but simultaneously I will be receiving wisdom and insights from my soul and guides, even the souls of the people I am engaging with physically or through the ether.

It can feel like a super-highway of messages at times, but once you get used to knowing the source of each message, it is fun to be the recipient of so many insights and foresights.

I say foresights, because sometimes I get warnings on what may arise soon. This is felt along with a sense of knowing – although the future can change from its current set of probabilities.

Of course, if I ask questions, I generally get answers as I tune in. I am often awoken in the middle of the night to receive downloads of key wisdom that a certain spirit or my own soul may want me to hear and process somehow. The downloads, for those who have not yet had them, feel like someone is tuning your brain like you would tune a radio. A kind of screech is also discernible. Sometimes you can determine what a download is giving you, but sometimes it can just be felt and not understood.

If you experience this, it's best to realise that the messages are just gifts of some kind from the universe that are designed to help you.

As I moved deeper into later phases of the Arc, I become more adept at managing this constant messaging, and now really love it.

Alchemy Takes Over

There can come a point in your journey that you reach a point of substantial purity. Your energy field or essence has been cleansed sufficiently to allow your heart to completely take over your being. In this place, the balance between your heart and mind reverses.

As you gradually open to your awakening process and allow it to unfold, you remove the barriers to being in connection with you soul and can receive its intelligence more clearly. There will come a point in your journey where your ego is so significantly dissolved that it no longer forms a barrier to the purity of your heart being a dominant energy of your being.

It's here that a form of alchemy can take place, with your soul taking complete control of your mind, field, and physical body.

This is an amazing experience, but somewhat abnormal. Your soul energy is now sending intelligence to your brain unimpeded. It is healing your body automatically where it can, and it is cleansing your energy field of its own accord and with your conscious intent. This is our natural way to live, once we are home in our hearts.

I had the experience of my mind being effectively rewired by my soul. The synaptic nerves in my brain were altered to allow a different flow of energy through my form – from the soul within me, through my body, and into my mind. Effectively my mind became more of a receiver of intelligence, rather than a storage unit for information and memories.

This rebuilding process was quite discombobulating for about a week, as I adapted to the repatterning or reminding of my mind. My mind did not like the experience of changing roles and becoming second in-charge, rather than the boss of me.

How has this changed me?

It has changed some of the things I enjoyed in life, like formal dancing that required me to remember steps, making that process less simple. However, it has also helped me receive intuitive information more easily and, in doing so, has enhanced my ability to be more effective with my writing, and to have greater presence in my interactions with others.

I also feel greater poise and composure in my whole form. I'm not quite sure yet where this will lead me with my future self-expression, but I know that will continue to unfold and probably change.

Physically, this alchemy has slowed down my ageing process and is allowing me to have a higher immunity to diseases. Many viruses and bacterial germs are low vibrational organisms. When your vibration is higher than theirs, you have a natural ability to overcome them as your energy fields can reject them, and your body can kill them if they enter your form.

I'm not sure how far this process will go, but I'm told that as you fully enter your light, this alchemic process also goes to new heights. I hope to discuss this in future books for interested readers.

This path to higher consciousness comes with many wonderful side-effects, many of which I'm sure I have yet to be fully graced with. This is not a right or an expectation that I hold but will be a privilege if it occurs more for me. This will be determined by the universe through my soul, not my mind.

The human mind is not fully utilised in most people. Science tells us that there are parts of our brain that are dormant. I understand that this alchemic process can open the unused chambers of the human mind and stimulate them to support our lives. From this you may develop new abilities and skills you never knew you had!

Ultimately, our minds and bodies can become far more highly evolved when they are receiving the energy of our eternal soul.

After experiencing this 'advanced normality', I would never want to go back to my old normal ways. I doubt I could anyway, even if I tried.

From here, we can align with one of the truths of the universe – that anything is possible when you believe it is, and you are living as the vibration of love!

Let the power of the Arc spark the illusions in your dark!

CHAPTER 22

Living in the Energies of Gratitude and Trust

Gratitude

When love aligns you with the energy of pure love that your soul offers, you will begin to feel more grateful of the sometimes-difficult experiences you encounter, and this is every being's natural state.

Once you understand how you are evolving, you can even love the process. It may sound counter-intuitive, but the process of welcoming pain because you know you will grow through it, is a powerful message to the universe that you are fully in the experiences coming forth, that you are committed and ready to be fully supported on your journey to your light.

This desire to expand will be met by a loving energy to assist you at a faster pace. You can dial up or down the intensity of the experiences that you are having, simply by asking for what you want. The universe is always present with you.

Through this omnipresence, the universe is always listening and cares for you, it loves to help you expand and grow. We are all universal beings, so in the long run we must. This will never change and can't be stopped, other than temporarily by the roadblocks that our egos put in the way.

However, our expansion will naturally be sped up when we are welcoming and learning from our intended lessons and are grateful for what is unfolding in your interests, unless you consciously ask it to be slowed down.

You will only ever be offered the learnings and experiences that you are ready for and are able to integrate into your being. So, the more enthusiastic you are to learn and grow, the more intense will be the lessons that are offered.

No quality teacher should ever offer you teachings that are beyond your existing consciousness or ability to receive a lesson's wisdom. You should be capable of handling the experiences and synchronicity that come forth for you, to step into and use to integrate your new awareness.

If you are given concepts and experiences before you are ready to hold them, the process would not provide you with clarity, but only serve to confuse you, effectively slowing down your progress along your path.

My experience with gratitude was a double-edged sword. I loved every opportunity I was provided to grow through; but, at the same time, I was initially quite impatient with my unfolding. I wanted it so badly, having experienced so many lifts in lightness after a lifetime of pain, that I wanted to get ahead of the natural process.

I tried too hard. I'm sure this led me to chase and experience several 'false dawns' that I did not need to witness.

Trying is not an energy that aligns with love, because love and control are opposites.

Effectively, my mind tried to take ownership and control of my awakening and thought it was my consciousness, which it is not. This energy of control took me away from love and into fear – the fear that I would fail to expand as fast as my ego wanted me to.

I was not in the energy of gratitude, because I was never fully satisfied with my progress, despite it being quite fast, according to my learned mentors. Despite being warned that this lack of gratitude could be an issue for me, and require me to repeat lessons, I still allowed my ego to take me down this rocky and winding path. I was a bit obsessive to my own detriment.

In hindsight, I did the best I could, given my consciousness levels, and am glad to say that I have now willingly handed my unfolding to my soul. That doesn't mean I am any less enthusiastic about my unfolding, it just means that I am now more in the energies of love and gratitude, particularly after going through the advanced purification process called the Dark Night of the Soul, which I discuss below.

I still love being my own bridge to new possibilities; but I recognise that my mind is not my bridge, just one of the pylons that support it.

Every day I ask my soul what my next lessons are and await the messages of love and related synchronicities. If there are no lessons arising that day, I accept that situation and relax.

This allowing energy is non-controlling, and more aligned with love. I love the new lessons I receive, but I don't chase lessons that are illusory, or which I am not ready to receive. That would be like a dog chasing a parked car.

As a result, I am more in flow and waste less energy on irrelevant diversions. There is a saying that, when you chase the dragon, you end up getting burnt. I think I did that on my path, and ended up trying to clear pain and suffering that was either not yet ready to be faced, or didn't truly exist. I went into dark caves I didn't need to be in and didn't find the light I was seeking. My mind did not grasp the concept that I would get the lessons I needed when I was ready to face them.

This was a form of distrust, and spiritual ego.

It can be hard to let go and trust your soul because, most likely, if you are like I was, this is a new concept that can take time for your mind to accept.

But I learned a valuable lesson that is now serving me well – to be patient. I have now slowed down to speed up.

I would love you to learn from my mistakes, to make your journey easier to navigate. I circumnavigated and went the long way around, whereas I could have navigated my way straight into the arms of nature!

Your higher consciousness will always grace you with its presence when you are ready for it, and you will slowly become more and more grateful that it is penetrating your being.

Trust

When we encounter disruption in our lives, it can be easy to lose trust in life. This is akin to losing trust in love, for all is ultimately love. Often this distrust is subconscious and manifests as gradual or subtle changes in the ways we think and behave.

Many of us learn not to trust ourselves at an early age and this can continue throughout our mature years. This is easy to do if we are subjected to strong control by those around us and are regularly forced to comply with the wishes of others. We begin to doubt our own judgements and ability to make legitimate choices. Strict parenting, schooling or work environments can be sources of this type of control.

Then, if loss or disruption occurs in our lives as we mature, despite our best efforts to do the 'right thing', we can start to lose trust in the world around us too. The result can be a life devoid of trust, both inward and outward. This can then lead us into the energy of withdrawal. Without high levels of trust of any form, we withdraw from aspects of life that have led us into past problems. The result can be a loss of opportunities. Once bitten twice shy, you might say!

Unfortunately, when you adopt the inner energy of withdrawal it will be met by the energy of withdrawal externally. This is often referred to as the Law of Attraction in spiritual writings. The result for many can be isolation or loneliness. We lock ourselves away repeatedly to stay safe. These behaviours are becoming increasingly common in modern society because of the high levels of competition, crime, and despair we witness on a regular basis. But remember, what we fear has a higher probability of coming true, for a fear is no more than a limiting belief, unless it is inherently based in wisdom not illusion!

I certainly experienced this situation after the repeated losses I outlined in earlier chapters. My trust in life was smashed and I wanted to escape from it and find safety alone for several years.

When I was ready to face it, I went inward first and, through the application of the Arc to my circumstances and feelings, was able to rebuild my belief structures so I could remerge and reconnect with life more fully. This process allowed me to ultimately face my core issue: a lack of trust in myself.

Since our inner reality always radiates out into our outer reality, it is important to restore this aspect of our psyche to be able to invite our full possibilities into reality. Distrust and withdrawal are not energies that are typically conducive to great levels of personal success, as they are birthed in the energy of fear, not love. In effect, we attract what we become.

Once we accept that we are the creators of our own realities, and all that happens to us allows us to grow, we can then start to rebuild our trust in love and life. Higher self-awareness opens the door to the more we truly seek.

The Arc can help anyone who has struggled with trust issues to step back into life with a renewed and positive attitude. It allows us to make more sense of our challenging and perhaps painful experiences. New beginnings beckon in these rekindled and natural energies.

Imagine a society with greater levels of trust because people have learned to trust in their own desires and decisions. Higher levels of sovereignty, with unity, will follow.

The Code of Happiness that I outlined in my book *Where Your Happiness Hides*, can then manifest on a wider scale. The result: a happier world full of happier people!

CHAPTER 23

Advanced Self-Awareness Experiences

Your Experience Is Always Unique

The following sections detail some advanced experiences that I encountered on my journey.

Please note, however, that none of the following should be seen as a guide to others as to what should happen or be done, because we are all different in terms of our evolution and vibration levels. I may have had more issues to work through than many readers, and been carrying greater conditioning and karma that had to be removed because of my energetic reactions to my past.

We all experience what we are ready for and needing to experience, to allow us to expand our personal consciousness. There are no rules here, as the universe is always dynamic in the way that it unfolds and is experienced for us all.

Those with naturally high vibrations or awareness may be ready for certain experiences earlier than I was.

Some of the younger generations may also have possibly been born into a less conditioned society. Some are purer of heart naturally. They may carry less karma for they have experienced less lives on Earth. This is why many are referred to as Crystal or Indigo Children in spiritual circles. Their vibrations are naturally high as they are here to lift the overall vibration of the Earth as we enter the realm of higher energies.

Transcendence

I encountered and became capable of transcending my limiting beliefs and attachments about eight years into my awakening. My ability to process new levels of self-awareness then changed as I expanded.

Originally, I worked primarily with my mind to expand, though it had limited impact because it did not have a great intersection with energy.

Then my body became the key processor, applying the kundalini energies (life force) within me, and eventually I was processing my learnings on all three levels – mind, body, and spirit (i.e. soul) simultaneously. This was an intense experience, but fast and effective.

Transcendence can take place when your connection to your soul strengthens. From my experience, it involves handing over the prevailing learning, or change in self-awareness, to your soul, and allowing it to control the release of your pain. It is a powerful experience and will enable you to process karmic energies from this and past lives.

The universe will never fully release the energy of an illusion that you have adopted in your egocentric mind until you have become completely, and I mean 100%, conscious of the lesson that you were meant to learn. In these circumstances, your new awareness can be processed through all levels of your being simultaneously.

In me, it begins instantly once I surrender. My mind, energy field and body all commence processing the releases I am enduring, together with the help of my chakras and the kundalini.

I personally view swirling energies above me in the shape of a tunnel, normally crimson in colour. The enlightened ones call it the Slipstream, and it is the universal vibrational energy that facilitates releases. My body usually shakes with the kundalini energy, and as my field shifts, the toxic energy cells in my form are immediately released. This comes out of my body as mucus, like you might get in a bacterial infection or virus. In me, this can last for up to three or four days.

From my experience, my body can take longer to integrate the shift, because it needs to release toxins that mirror my old, outdated sources of awareness through its physical systems.

This release is reliant on the organs and systems in the body that manage toxic releases, such as the kidneys, lungs, urinary system, liver, skin, and so on, to allow the toxins to pass back to nature. The effectiveness of these organs and the associated toxic releases are influenced by the health of your body, and the lifestyle choices that you make.

Sleep and water are important inputs to speed up this process. Being in nature generally speeds up the process too, as it allows energies to flow from the energy field in an accelerated way.

By releasing toxic cells from our bodies in this way, the soul allows more space for light to enter. The cells of the human body mirror the energies within the human energy field. If you change your field or essence, through the attainment of higher self-awareness, your whole being shifts, including your cellular structure. This makes you lighter – as it must, for you are a whole being.

I wouldn't ask your local doctor about this. From my experiences it's not in the vocabulary of modern medicine – yet!

Transcendence, however, as it occurs for an individual, is an advanced process. Prior to transcendence being possible within you, you are likely to experience partial releases of toxic energies. These will continue to return for further releases in different ways as your vibration continues to rise.

They may also present themselves in different chakras at different points of your awakening for release. You will only get the releases you are ready for, because they match your vibrational energy levels.

Transcendence is different to Transcendental Meditation. The latter involves the repetition of a mantra or sound, like a chant, to promote relaxation, stress release, and higher states of consciousness.

There are many other differing practices or modalities to stimulate change and awareness within you. They will serve to lift your vibration and conscious awareness if you allow them to, but will not remove significant karmas unless the respondent also seeks to learn the lessons that are on offer in that experience. This is a core component of the journey to higher consciousness.

The Dark Night of the Soul

There is much information in spiritual books about what is sometimes called the long or 'dark night of the soul'. Other experts have referred to it as the death of the ego or going through the eye of the needle.

Each of these descriptions refers to an advanced purification or transcendence process that occurs before a person can finally enter their light. It is often marked by a strong sense of confusion, a sense of total helplessness, stagnation of the human will, and a deep feeling that you have been abandoned by life, and therefore by God. In this experience, you are likely to question the meaning of your life.

In this process, the ego finally succumbs to the soul and gives up its need to control your awakening and life. It dissolves into your wholeness. Darkness steps out and light steps in.

As we go along the path to higher conscious awareness, we generally expand as different limiting beliefs and attachments are recognised and partially surrendered to. However, the extent to which we truly transcend these energies, each time they arise, is predicated on the level of surrender with which we approach them. In other words, the extent to which we process them – in the purity of love in our hearts, or the ego that resides in our minds – and claims every piece of new awareness as its own achievement.

I faced my realisations multiple times as I evolved along my path, and my vibration gradually rose as a result. However, dealing with issues repeatedly was confusing and frustrating to say the least. However, it was not until I aligned with the vibration of love within myself and I totally surrendered to the pain I felt within me, that I entered this dark night of the soul experience.

It was a crushing feeling to go through, and as I traversed it there were times when I would have been happy to die, such was the sense of complete despair that I felt. I cried with a potency that I had never experienced before, and my body shook uncontrollably. In fact, I struggled to recognise my own sounds as I cried and collapsed into my pain. It was a brutal experience. This went on for weeks.

I'm sure everyone who faces this process has a different experience, but in the end, I eventually entered a deep realisation that, no matter what happens in my life, I am and was always loved by God and by my own soul. Therefore, no matter what I had ever seemingly failed or succeeded at, it was of no real consequence, because loving my life and feeling fulfilled was all that really mattered.

My ego had stepped aside in my floods of tears and pain and surrendered to love. It finally gave up believing that it was the origin and orchestrator of my conscious awareness. Finally the truth sank in, in a blaze of pain. But to get there, I had to allow love and the wisdom in my pain to totally overwhelm and take control of me.

Humanity is obsessed by the need to avoid failure. It is a deep and core fear that controls and constrains many of us.

I was no different in my life, and every time I supposedly failed, I struggled to find self-compassion and self-forgiveness within me.

Accordingly, we seek our own mind-based version of success to avoid opening to the pain of failure.

The Dark Night of the Soul allowed me to feel into and dismiss concepts of success and failure from my psyche and to see that, at the end of the day, love and happiness is truly all the matters in life. I realised that I could never really fail or succeed, for they are both just masks of the ego that I was taught to wear, and they are merely created by expectation rather than reality.

If you are truly *loved* by God and an important aspect of the universe, *can* you ever truly fail?

The truth that I came to feel in this peak moment of darkness was that I truly cannot fail – ever. I know my life will never be the same again after this natural but painful experience!

The experience also allowed me to see, uncategorically, that my soul is the only source of my higher conscious awareness. It has unlimited intelligence and power to create. My mind had controlled large aspects of my enlightenment process, and the Dark Night of the Soul allowed me to witness how fanciful it was to allow such a limited apparatus as my mind, to take me beyond the third dimensional version of consciousness. It was the peak experience in which I was able to surrender to the God-essence within me. Finally, life was living me, not the other way around.

One of the hardest experiences of my life has taken me a step closer to knowing my light. Now I had to let go fully, focus on having fun and hand my awakening over to God.

Ascension

Ascension, as a word, describes a form of rising or becoming more elevated. Forty days after the death of Jesus Christ, he *ascended* into heaven to be with the Father, or God.

While we all have the potential to *ascend* in the same way, a soul can only ascend after it has mastered all the lessons it was intended to overcome on Earth, is no longer subject to the Earth's karmic cycle, and is no longer required to return to Earth to rebalance further karmic energies.

Of course, once a soul has ascended, it may later choose to return to Earth for other purposes, including just enjoying being in physical form, or perhaps bringing important wisdom to the Earth.

For those who choose to face their karmic debts now, the karmic cycle can now come to an end, as higher vibrational light energies currently present upon the planet are offering us all the opportunity to evolve from the third to at least the fifth dimension in this incarnation.

For those who do not choose to face their karma, they will continue to experience the density of a third dimensional life, reincarnating into subsequent lives until this is mastered.

The fifth dimension is of a higher vibration and therefore occupied only by beings that have risen beyond the third dimension to live from a place of unconditional love.

In the fifth and higher dimensions, beings can have advanced capabilities and can, among other things, manifest from love, remember their concurrent lives, communicate telepathically, and transcend time and space. These beings are fully connected to their universal selves and, in turn, all things. The movie franchise *Star Wars* calls this kind of energy, the Force.

Thus, while the concept of transcendence involves going through and above something, ascension refers to the evolutionary process of having experienced universal love, then going beyond the vibration of the third dimension on the Earth plane.

It has long been recorded as occurring at a human's time of death, such as the Bible detailing Jesus 'rising' 40 days after his crucifixion. He died and subsequently ascended. Not that he needed to die to ascend, I suspect!

Jesus came to Earth to bring a message of light. In doing so, he achieved many miracles, including healing people. When he walked the Earth, he was already free of any third dimensional density, and was living from the energy of his soul, a place of unconditional love, with his ego dissolved into his wholeness. This was most likely true for other beings such as Buddha, Saint Germain, Ramana and so on, who are now referred to as Ascended Masters.

The energy of universal love can also take you beyond and into other high vibrational energies, like light and others that I have yet to encounter. In the purity of the metaphysical, your soul is not encumbered by the density of being encapsulated in a physical body and a 3D world.

Kundalini Energy

The kundalini is a natural energy force within the human body that is associated with your life force. It has healing powers. It is known to traverse your body, often through the chakras and your spinal cord. The kundalini is often represented in pictorial form as a coiled snake. In most human beings, kundalini energy lies dormant and unused near the base of their spine.

There are different ways to activate the kundalini within you. Of course, in some it may be naturally active, but this is rare. *These are the two I have experienced:*

- *Kundalini Yoga – this is a form of yoga used to stimulate the kundalini energy within your body. It would appeal to any yoga lovers. I did it for a few months, but found it very physically demanding; and,*
- *Kundalini Activation – there are gifted people who can activate the kundalini within you by just placing their hands above you and introducing an activating energy into your body. The process is normally accompanied by loud music, since music is a form of light. Being a vibration, it is known to bring forth the activation activity.*

I found the kundalini activation process to be highly effective in my case. It took about 30 minutes, though the time it takes to activate a person's kundalini can vary significantly. Resistance in the mind can slow down the process.

I did it about 10 times, and each time was an incredible experience that made my whole-body shake. Emotions arose and my chakras within me reacted powerfully. I learned a lot about the pain I was holding onto, and was able to grow in consciousness as a result. I also felt much lighter after each session as toxic energies were released, and my conscious awareness expanded.

I witnessed many different responses by other participants too; which included shaking, dancing, crying, screaming, and laughing. It may sound harsh and unpleasant, but it is just the body releasing toxic energies through the power of your own life force.

I recommend it to all those on the journey to higher consciousness. It helped in my application of the Arc and my participation in other modalities.

The Mystical Merkabah

We all have a Merkabah within our energetic structures. Like the kundalini energies, this energy has been largely forgotten by the modern world, and therefore the Merkabah is dormant in most of us, with its power substantially lost to most. However, many spiritual people are rediscovering it and having theirs activated.

The word Merkabah is Hebrew for chariot, for it is referred to in scriptures and ancient writings as the Chariot of God. The Merkabah symbol is comprised of two intersecting tetrahedrons (i.e. like pyramids) that spin in opposite directions, creating a three-dimensional energy field within our human energy fields. It is centred in the human field in the heart chakra, the centre of our being.

The Merkabah allows your consciousness to return to higher dimensions, and its activation is therefore critical if you want to take your conscious awareness beyond the third dimension in which we physically live and connect to other dimensions.

Its existence has long been denied by established institutions, like governments and religions, as they have known for centuries about the power this would give a population with active Merkabahs.

Many people involved in modern establishments would, however, no longer understand the Merkabah and its power.

The Merkabah is said to be so powerful that, when a person's Merkabah is fully active, it is visible on a radar screen, and it can alter weather patterns in that person's immediate vicinity.

The patron of the Merkabah in the spirit realm is Archangel Metatron. His energy can establish any connection in the universe, as it has unlimited power. If you activate your Merkabah, you can call upon him to assist in this process.

In 2019, I attended a course about the Merkabah and was able to activate my Merkabah. It only took me about 30 minutes to do this through deep meditation and the power of intention, but its impact on my life has been profound. It has assisted me to have many incredible metaphysical experiences, and I will never forget the feeling of it opening, as energy rushed into and out of my field.

I would urge all those on a deep awareness or spiritual path, to research this opportunity and consider opening your Merkabah.

A Diversity of Awareness Generating Modalities

Becoming more advanced through 'spiritual' or awareness activities can assist your journey to higher consciousness, particularly if you take part in them as you journey through the Arc.

These modalities serve to lift your vibration by disarming your ego, and allowing you enhanced access to your soul and universal energies. They give you the opportunity to raise your self-awareness and bring your accumulated karmas and pain to light.

Some of the modalities include:

- Reiki energy healing,
- Sound healings, including Solfeggio frequencies,
- Kundalini yoga and activation,

- Spiritual medicines such as mushrooms, cactus and Ayahuasca,
- Ice-baths,
- Different forms of meditation,
- Crystal healing,
- Ecstatic dance,
- Theta Healing,
- Breathwork,
- Cacao ceremonies,
- Pranic healing,
- Channelling Universal Wisdom,
- Past life karmic releases,
- Yoga,
- Tantric lovemaking,
- Floating, and
- Accessing the Akashic Records.

All of these modalities, and more, can be researched on the internet. They are all consistent with and can be done in conjunction with the Arc.

I have done many of these modalities to assist my awakening.

Indeed, should you apply any of these modalities to your own journey, it is vital that you identify and explore any lessons possible in the energies and emotions arising during the application. Understand them fully, and the issues that come to light can be partially or fully transcended.

Past Life Karmic Removal

Most of us have had multiple lives on the Earth. We have been born and experienced death many times over. I say *most* because many beings can, at any time, be having their first life on Earth.

The karmic cycle has been real for centuries and persists today for most souls on Earth.

I have been through approximately 60 of my 'past lives', using different approaches to know them and remove any related karmic energies.

These included:

- *Accessing past lives with a respected psychic and three Body Talk specialists.*
- *Accessing the Akashic Records through my own meditations and witnessing them unfold.*
- *Travelling to places on Earth where I have had past lives, to allow them to be removed by my soul. I did this in Egypt, Hawaii, central Australia, and the United Kingdom, at multiple sites where I know I once lived. I was guided to them by higher beings.*
- *Discussing relevant past lives directly with higher beings in metaphysical channels.*
- *Undertaking a series of sessions with an expert in human energy fields and karmic removal.*

I asked only for information about past lives that served me significantly in my expansion activities and aligned with my personal challenges in this life.

Many of the major limiting beliefs I encountered in this life had their genesis in past experiences on this planet. By shifting those beliefs through my past lives, I have been able to negate the associated energy and pain that was manifesting in this life.

Dealing with similar issues in this life then allowed me to also change the energy of past experiences, as well as assisting any souls who experienced those karmic events with me.

To my surprise, several people I knew in this life, and still interact with, had been a party to my karmic experiences in centuries past!

The pain we carry in this life can be derived from this life or from past lives. It may have no logical explanation because we have carried it into this life for clearing. It may even impact on our health, for the energy associated with this karma can be trapped in our energy fields and in our existing bodies.

Working with my karmic energy specialist has been fascinating, because it has shown me how deeply I need to fully understand the lessons behind my karma, and be able to articulate the 'pay-offs' and 'rip-offs' associated with that karma in this life, and the associated beliefs and energies I have held as a result. This articulation has taken hours, at times, because of its complexity.

By 'rip-off', I mean what these energies have cost me in this life.

By 'pay-off', I mean how my ego has used them to protect and project me in this life.

Taking away the karma instantly alters what is possible while we are still alive, for it raises our vibration and purifies our energy fields, minds and bodies.

It has altered my energy field and, in turn, my cellular structure for the better.

Releasing past karmas may not be of interest to some readers, though it can be done simultaneously to eliminate current life traumas and pain. Karmic patterning resulting from the past can influence our current life experiences. It can be released when we have an understanding of the originating event and are ready to forgive all involved and let go.

The removal of past life karma is advanced, and to do it effectively you may need the help of souls who are highly connected in the first instance. As your consciousness advances, you will most likely be able to do it yourself, and fast.

I started my karmic removal work when I was entering Phase 3 of the Arc. I'm now in Phase 9 and still doing it. I think it's fun!

Tantric Lovemaking

For two years, I had the opportunity to study and experience tantric lovemaking. I explored this in books, at conferences, and by being mentored by two lovely woman who helped me with private coaching.

All this exploration showed me how much humanity has lost touch with what is possible when two lovers make love on a more conscious level. There are learned people in the world who understand these principles, and apply them in their daily lives, though they are in the minority of aware souls.

Tantra takes lovemaking to a more energetic and soul-based level. Most sexual activity expressed in Western society is extremely physical. It involves much friction between the bodies of two lovers. It is also focussed on touching and genital expression.

Tantra adds in the power of breathing, eye-gazing, and the transfer of life force energy between two people through the chakra systems of the body. It is less about genital orgasm, and more about facilitating orgasms on a broader scale throughout the body, through the entire chakra system. Those who are adept at it experience lovemaking that lasts for many hours, and orgasms that can last for 20 to 40 minutes.

Tantric sex is more difficult for men to master than women, because it requires men to maintain erections for longer periods of time, without any normal orgasm taking place. Women are superior sexually to men, as a rule, because they can orgasm multiple times in a sexual experience. Women adapt very quickly to Tantric sex because of this gift. Tantra can give a man greater sexual prowess and allow them to match the sexual power of their partner.

Many people have become somewhat blocked from expressing and radiating their sexual energy out into the world. This has its genesis in thousands of years of conditioned thinking, which has taught us that the free expression of sexual energy is somewhat undesirable, unless it is applied in a close relationship, like a marriage. Some religions have reinforced this unnatural belief structure.

I was brought up with this conditioned way of thinking in the 1960s and 1970s. It held me back from getting involved in many pleasurable physical experiences in my life.

We need to understand that we live in a physical dimension and lovemaking is one of the greatest gifts we can experience in this dimension. Tantra facilitates a very special experience, though it is probably more suited to situations where two people have a deep soul-to-soul connection, not just a physically dominated connection. It is less adaptable to casual sexual interludes because love is, at its core, not just lust. It is also typically performed over extended periods of time, typically multiple hours.

Tantric sex is extremely intimate and touches the souls of those involved. It can also bring forth pain and emotional healings by virtue of the deep energetic connections that can arise. This can effectively support anyone on a quest to find higher self-awareness through their own arc of personal transformation.

Although I am yet to apply what I have learned about Tantra in a profound personal relationship, I have experienced enough to understand how incredible the gift of Tantra can bring to interactions between two lovers.

It is a shame that this natural art of making love has been extracted from the sexual vocabulary of mainstream sexual expression.

Tantra is a form of lovemaking between two hearts, who feel deeply for each other. It serves to open your energetic systems, including your chakra systems, and can be the source of much joy for those with the skills and desire to do it. Experienced in full love and integrity, it has been known to connect both individuals to their full light.

There is much on the internet and in bookshops if you want to explore it further. Your partner and relationship may flourish even more once you understand what is truly natural and possible in the bedroom!

The art of Tantra should not be reserved for the minority who are more spiritually orientated. This is a gift for us all to enjoy and benefit from, during our incarnations on Earth.

Telepathy

For much of my life I believed that telepathy was a way of reading people's minds. My personal experiences have now shown that this is not the case.

As my energetic abilities have expanded, I have learned that I can speak to the souls of others through the ether. I can send them messages and receive messages from the souls of others too, including the souls of the deceased.

Minds cannot operate through the ether, only souls can, because all souls in the universe are intrinsically connected. Our minds can be involved in telepathy as an interpreter and organiser, but no more.

Telepathy can be a much purer way to get a message to another because their conditioned minds do not tamper with any messages sent.

The ability of all souls to connect with each other, even after death, has no limits. They can choose not to do so if an energetic connection is felt to be inappropriate by the receiving soul.

I once had a relationship with a highly evolved woman, and we could sense into each other's feelings, send each other sexual energy, and experience our respective physical pains from thousands of kilometres away. We could send each other visions and alter them through the ether together. Our connection was extraordinary.

I often receive messages from those who have passed, either for myself or to give to family and friends. I do not seek these, but I do trust them when they come to me.

As you become more conscious by applying the Arc, or any other process to higher self-awareness, including your own natural abilities and intuition, you will naturally increase your vibration or sense of lightness. This can bring forth metaphysical abilities commensurate with your new levels of consciousness.

I had no such experiences until my mid-50s, but they have continued to expand as I have moved through the Arc and into higher phases. I am not yet sure how far this will take me, but I am truly fascinated to find out!

Channelling Universal Wisdom

I have done a lot of work with metaphysical beings to broaden my horizons and help me develop the Arc. This exposure has taken place through several modalities, not dissimilar to the list above.

The most significant modality that has helped me through my journey has been channelling sessions that have directly connected me to universal wisdom. I stumbled upon this process through synchronicity, but many conversations with major metaphysical beings over a seven-year period have helped me find greater self-awareness and wisdom.

They do not tell me answers as a rule, but they give me guidance as to what I need to consider next on my path. They have also given me challenges to take on. To date, I have had hundreds of these types of conversations, which would amount to thousands of hours of interactions with pure intelligence. This is a key source of wisdom, from which I have been able to write this book and to expand personally.

I have held conversations with beings such as:

- Mary Magdalene,
- St Germain,
- Archangel Michael,
- Archangel Metatron,
- Jesus Christ,
- Thoth,

- Ramana,
- Mary, Mother of God,
- Horus,
- Osiris,
- Mother Nature, and
- Many, many others!

I consider access to these great beings to be a great privilege.

This book would not have been possible without their loving guidance to stimulate my curiosity and enquiries about the truths of life, and the path to higher consciousness.

Life Reviews Before Death

When you die, you are given a life review in the metaphysical realm, let's call it heaven, to clarify what you have learned in this life and what you may need to readdress in a 'future' life. This process untethers you from the Earth and allows your spirit to rest and be free in the metaphysical realm.

It is possible to undertake this review before you die, to free you from any attachments you may have to aspects and elements of your Earthly experiences. This can detach your consciousness from the physical and give you greater capacity to consciously experience the metaphysical realm before you are deceased.

I have undergone this process. It was intense, taking over 15 hours of work with an expert, with metaphysical beings present. Again, this is an advanced process, and I was not considered ready for it by my soul until I entered Phase 9 of the Arc.

There are many advanced aspects and modalities that you can activate and use to assist your journey to higher consciousness. Many religious organisations are unable to teach people about them, for they have been forgotten through centuries of conditioned thinking. But there are gifted souls out there who can. If you want to get involved with any of them, the choice is yours.

These advanced forms of activation are no substitute for being consciously aware of your passage through evolution, and the reality that truth and love are found in the self-awareness that lies inside you already. However, they give you great assistance on your path as you step onto it and progress through your awakening process.

Instant Awakenings

There are recorded cases of people experiencing what are known as Instant Awakenings. In these situations, a person connects directly to their universal self and goes straight to being in the energy of source.

Obviously, if this occurs, a person does not need to go through the experience of working through their limited beliefs, fears, and karmic energies, and aligning with the vibration of their true selves to find the universal love that lies within them.

All is possible in the incredible universe to which we belong. Accordingly, this kind of shift, although extremely rare, is possible if an individual's soul deems it appropriate.

Like most people on their awakening journey, I did not experience this type of instant transformation, so I cannot describe it with any authority. However, the process I have experienced has allowed me to expand my conscious awareness gradually, and in turn remember and share the wisdom of the Arc. For this I am eternally grateful.

RETURNING HOME

CHAPTER 24

Remembering What You Already Are

Beliefs Give Way to Knowing

The pathway to higher consciousness can be hard and challenging. It will encourage you to face your 'demons' and limiting beliefs. It will require great courage to turn and face your pain, and to dispel the many illusions that once limited and defined your life. It's not for the faint-hearted, even though it is the medicine that a faint heart truly desires. The awakening process 'rips you open', purifies you and gives you the opportunity to expand your conscious awareness. It's a magical journey of self-discovery.

How many purification processes do you know of that are not messy, for they involve the extraction of toxicity and density in most cases.

But as you progress, you will come to witness this natural process for the paradox it truly is.

On the one hand, you had to climb the mountain to see the majestic views, and the Arc gave you the strength to illuminate your ascending path. At the same time, when you look back sometimes, you can recognise that all your life you've felt uneasy, sensing that something was missing, that your life was somehow incomplete. Slowly, you can now see that you've been trying to fill this nagging hole, and its hollow sense of doubt, with things outside of yourself. But it never seemed to be enough. You never felt like you were enough. Something was never quite right. Even though you were doing what you had been taught to do, even though you just kept trying, hoping for more. It felt like a constant loop you couldn't quite escape from.

You therefore start to feel sad that you've spent most of your life trying to prove to yourself, and the world, that you were worth loving. All that trying to be important and admired, struggling to be noticed, competing to win, pushing through your pain, obsessing over what you owned or had lost, regretting that great love that got away – all falls away in a sudden epiphany of knowing...

Finally, the truth burns inside you, when you least expected it to, when you wondered if all this soul-searching you've committed to, and the pain it brought forth to face, was worth it. Suddenly, your beliefs give way to this knowing...

That it was all without meaning, that other life. That this new life is all that matters, for it feels like home.

As your fears melt away, a bridge to the new you appears from behind the mist and you know that it's time to cross over into a new paradigm. Your rebirth is upon you, and you didn't need to physically die to find it, you just needed to search inside your soul and allow your ego to dissolve to know what you always were – pure love, living a human life!

The love you had been searching for was always inside you, you just didn't know it until now.

Now you need nothing, because you finally see that you had everything you truly ever needed. Love is all that matters, and you are it. God loves you completely. What more could you need?

The knowing inside you grows and finds its confidence: that you are enough and always were.

Your life will never be the same again. Now you can participate in life with a different intent, and a different agenda – to just have fun, be fulfilled and create a beautiful life. How others judge you no longer matters!

And all it took was for you to stop believing in illusions and start remembering the truth in your heart.

You need nothing to be loved because you already are, so why not have a really good time as the true and wonderful you?

You ARE the Outcome You Seek Already

One of the hardest moments in your awakening journey arises when you witness a great truth emerge for you and from within your consciousness. On your path, you will have encountered many powerful and emotional moments as you confront your truths. However, as hard as you try to reach your full light, there comes a point where reality sets in. No matter what truths you encounter and realisations you intersect with, at some point you will see that the ego cannot ever take you to full enlightenment.

This is a confronting realisation because you now know that you can do no more than invite the experience you seek to come forth. You now understand that all control is irrelevant. Your thoughts matter not; your experiences through feeling are everything.

Your ego is not capable of the energy that your eternal soul already is. It has played a valuable role in assisting with the process of discovering all you needed to meet and all that stood in your way. The Arc has helped you to move to higher levels of consciousness and to prepare for what you seek. It has given you a platform to move away from thought and into knowing, from pain to possibility. The universe has witnessed your commitment, but the universe is in control, not you. The will of God is ultimately the determining factor.

You are collapsing into the awareness that your pure consciousness cannot be achieved like other goals you may have set in your life, yet it is the key step to the final discovery of your holy grail becoming possible.

When you relax, immerse yourself in the full awareness of your inner sense and allow your ego to dissolve, you are finally ready for your true self to burst forth, through you and for you, beyond the boundaries of your mind. The Dark Night of the Soul is often the fulcrum for this important realisation to grace your path, as it crushes your ego and gets it out of the way.

By identifying your limiting beliefs and all the density you have been living within, you bring forth all that needs to be brought into the light, through the doorway of pain. Opening to this reality allows you to move through this incredible and natural transformation, which you have chosen to participate in, and to fully activate the divinity that you are, and the divinity codes that were previously dormant within your being. The normal resistance you once subconsciously honoured is on the run!

This is where the full magic can explode from within you. It's here that your full truth can now become you. You have reached and knocked on the door to your true home – but only God can decide when that door will burst open, so you can re-enter.

Your Extraordinary, Ordinary Life Arises

As human beings we are all mortal, and therefore temporary by nature in our current incarnations. This makes us all somewhat ordinary, or similar, on a physical level; although the human body is of course truly a miracle, like all of nature.

Still, it is a special choice to become our divine truth, a choice few people truly know about or make. Embracing your awakening with authenticity and advancing step by step to knowing your divine or true self, is not normal in this world at present. It is largely beyond mainstream thinking. However, for those who experience it, the extraordinary, ordinary or advanced normality awaits.

The opportunity to start again with fresh perspectives, and to live from the higher intelligence in your soul, is a gift that awaits those who choose to take this magical path. You can choose to apply this potent new energy to your existing life or use it to challenge yourself in ways that you never previously allowed yourself to pursue. Either choice is valid.

What if you could have that career that you always dreamt about, or the abundance and flow of money you previously thought was only for others? What if you could have higher levels of fun and fulfilment in everything you did? What if pain was a fleeting experience and adventure was your everyday way of being? What if true love with the partner of your dreams was your everyday experience of life?

Where your true self will take you, once you remember your connection to it, is impossible to know in advance. Only your divine self has that answer. However, if a life with less fear – freed of the limitations imposed on it by your old, entrenched reference points – sounds interesting and inspiring to you, why not choose the journey that the Arc can guide you through?

When you are fully connected to your heart, you are safe in knowing that, in every moment of your life, you will know what is in your own best interests. You can step forward into many exciting opportunities in which you will love to participate.

It doesn't give you control over your future or certainty of any particular outcomes, but it gives you the means to make wiser choices from the energy of love when you encounter the crossroads that will inevitably grace your path, be they big or small. Without access to this higher consciousness awareness, you are likely to make decisions to meet the expectations of your conditioned thoughts, and again encounter pain.

Why not let pain melt into possibility? It can, in the flame of truth.

This is the gift that connecting to your soul allows.

If you use the Arc, it can take you all the way home to a miraculous epiphany of truth, and a better experience of being you. Why not cross this bridge?

Love is the natural vibration of our future, for that is the will of

God. It is truly unstoppable. How would you like to be at the forefront of this dynamic transformational shift?

CONCLUDING REMARKS

CHAPTER 25

The Mystical Quest

Knowing Yourself is the Ultimate Destination

Knowing thyself has been described as the holy grail in legends passed down through the centuries for good reason. It allows truths, mysteries and higher intelligence to arise from within you that you may not have thought were possible.

Once you remember your truth by embarking on this journey, you will never want to return to your previous life of limited self-awareness. It will no longer be bearable by you.

However, as I mentioned in my introduction, the need to discover your true self is growing in its importance in our world. The world is an energetic experience for us all, and this experience is shifting. There is an energetic blending taking place as we enter a phase of higher vibration. Some are calling this higher vibrational world, the New Earth. As this energy gradually rises, you will not be able to be in the old ego-based energy of yourself that has been previously typical of the third dimension, without experiencing more suffering.

The only way to shift and move with the new energies is to let go of your conditioned ideas, and to evolve THROUGH your true self. The frequency and intelligence of yourself knows your future and why you are here on the Earth now. Your ego does not.

To become your embodied true self, you must bring your awareness to it as often as you can and meet the truth of what you really are. This will require you to go beyond thought into the experience of knowing yourself and the vibration of your soul. This is a practical process that you need to action again and again and again.

To find your true self and your light will challenge you to let go of all that you think you are, to release and stop developing your personality so that you can fully surrender to the eternal energy within you that knows the frequency at which you need to be for the future.

The Arc gives you a model to apply to help you move into this practice until it becomes automatic, and you surrender to your light and its wonderful powers and wisdom.

The Arc is ultimately about love and truth. Your truth is God's truth, and it lives in your soul. Each time you apply the Arc, you will venture gradually through it. Eventually, with enough practice, you will arrive at the gates of Phase 9 and allow yourself to experience your full activation. The time it takes you to master this process is not important, for there is no race to the gates of heaven. We will all get there in the end. In fact, we are already there. We are just having a holiday from heaven in a physical body!

By following the Arc, however, you can transcend the current epidemic of mental health issues, constantly worrying about your image, wealth, reputation or appearances. True safety and peace lie in our hearts and embodied self-awareness, and in replacing the concept of pain management with pain consciousness. The self is the eternal loving part of you, and unless you connect to it and feel its loving power, you are unlikely to ever know the full force of your true *self*.

When you allow this connection to self to be felt, great mysteries can arise from within you. This may include new levels of self-confidence, metaphysical abilities previously unknown to you, a new sense of purpose, and a deeper ability to love. You will undoubtedly refocus your life onto finding fulfilment, and drop many of the fears that kept you obsessed with concepts of fear and failure.

The application of the Arc to your life and the extent of the transformation possible has no limits, just like the universe of which we are a part. You may wish to apply it in certain circumstance, or in every experience of your life – good or bad. It is up to you and, no matter what you choose to do, you will benefit either way. Every lift, no matter how small, matters and should be celebrated.

Once you open the doorway to higher consciousness, you are unlikely to ever want to close it. Feeling lighter and more inspired, without artificially inducing it or just thinking it, can be addictive!

As you apply the Arc to your life and release old habits, addictions, limiting beliefs, egoic attachments and unhealthy relationships, the way you experience yourself will shift for the better. Even if your life circumstances don't change as fast as you may want, the way you feel about them will be more positive, for you will be witnessing them from a place of love not fear. Then, as you step into the opportunities arising from your new consciousness and the love in your heart, your life can't help but improve in the ways you intend. All is energy, after all. So, when you change your energy, you will change the energy of your third dimensional life. That's just how energetic connection naturally works.

Manifesting from the heart is far more potent than from the mind, because something manifested out of love has divine support behind it. It is therefore likely to be sustainable and well supported, even by the energy of money.

The universe is infinitely intelligent, and it knows everything you are doing, thinking, and always believing. You cannot hide from a source that has unlimited awareness, and also resides within you! Tell a lie and it relays it to the universe, for it is fully connected to all things. Tell a lie about another soul and that other soul knows you have done so. You are truly *always* connected to universal energies. It knows you better than you know you.

Aligning your heart, mind and body in the way nature intended is a powerful way to live. It allows you to unfold in-line with your divine intentions and plans. When you access your heart and feel through your body all your actions and thoughts can align with love. You will indeed become far more able to create what you want and love in your life. Living from love will bring you enhanced joy and fulfilment.

The veil that currently stands between your thoughts and your true desires in life, represents as low vibrational energies that link to unhelpful belief structures, including fears. Remove these and the creator within you can step forward and manifest new horizons for you to witness and pursue to your heart's content. Once unleashed, this creative energy will assist you to bring forth what was truly intended in your life.

Leave this to your conditioned mind, and the experiences you have will be quite different. Out of conditioned ignorance, most people try to live like someone else, perceiving their lives to be preferable. This is not a winning strategy, because everyone else's lives are already taken! This is the source of much pain in our lives because, deep within you, you know that you are being inauthentic in your attempts to be you. To some extent, you are a fake you.

I urge you to be true to you, and to live from the purity of your heart.

Those who need nothing (but love) get everything (for love is ultimately the source of everything in this amazing universe), and you can enjoy the reality of this wisdom by using the Arc to help you discover what took me years to remember.

It has worked wonders for me and turned my life from worry to wonder.

Those who can connect to their own source of love and truth, and trust in its messages, will have the ability to choose the life they want. The true God within you makes this possible.

May Your True Secrets Burst Forth

You can never be aware of a secret until it is in your awareness!

As you conclude this book, I hope you ponder the following concepts that your mind may reject, but your soul will not:

- Higher consciousness is the birthright of all. It is not just for selected beings. We are all equal.
- You are both metaphysical and physical. You are connected to both and recognising this is important to your life.
- Your pain and feelings are your passageway to higher consciousness. They will lead you home to your truth, if you let them teach you the wisdom you need to hear. You can learn from joy, but this is far less common.
- Emotions are just energies needing to be put in motion. When we let it go, we are free to make new choices unencumbered by the past. This creates infinite possibilities in our lives.
- You get what you need in life before you get what you truly want. Essentially therefore, those who need nothing, but love get everything in the end. Our egos are the enemies of this paradigm gracing our lives.
- You have a life path that you chose before you were born. By ignoring your heart, you ignore what your heart desires and you risk rewriting the divine story you have already written.
- Living from love opens the doorway to avoid suffering and become the true-you.
- Love and self-love can only ever be felt, not thought. Our world is awash with the thought of love and true love has become a true myth for most.
- The mystical state of being the true-you awaits you, if you do the work to attain higher consciousness. But beware this can be challenging.
- Self-awareness can generate awareness, not the other way around; but self-awareness can only ever be felt, not thought.
- Your true self is already within you. Your role is to allow it to clear away the pain, illusions and debris that keeps you separated from it.

- Anyone who connects totally to their heart through feeling, is likely to develop skills and abilities way beyond their comprehension. These mysteries will arise within you as you align with your truth, and you will find them astonishing.
- You are here to return to your truth, which is love; to evolve, just like the universe of which you are an important part. As you expand your awareness you can't help but create a wonderful experience of life for you to enjoy.
- Your real home is in your heart. It's the safest place you can live within. Trusting it is the gateway to complete bliss, a bliss you've probably never felt before in this life. Let love take you to your light, for here is your eternal home. Here you can rest in peace, while you are still a human being.
- The universe is ever expanding through love to new possibilities, as are you.
- All that happens in your life happens for you and through you, not to you. All has purpose. The infinite intelligence of your soul is always by your side and loving you through life. Here lies a great freedom once you surrender to this reality.
- All is a choice. The truths in this book have been unashamedly sourced from universal wisdom. What you do with this wisdom is totally up to you. But please ask your heart what it recommends you do, before you make that choice!

Your soul knows how to be the real you, and to discover the life you really want. It is urging you to allow it, to remind your mind of what and who you really are. You have the means to find your way home to the 'holy grail' that sits inside your heart; you have held this golden challis many times before and drunk from its purity. It's time to remember this destination while you are still alive on this planet. Your opportunity to choose it, and commit to the path that will unfold before you, is now upon you.

You are much more than you realise, and new beginnings await. Let your reality show you this more. By becoming more conscious, you have a far greater opportunity to choose the life that you want to live and fill your heart with joy. And all because you chose to face your pain and embrace new possibilities that you weren't even aware were on your destiny path.

I have been in full integrity and vulnerability in writing this book, as I had to be. The messages I bring to the world are true, yet contrary to mainstream thinking; so I know many will strive to strike them down, as is their valid choice to do so. I respect the choices of all my readers.

If you have reached this far into the book, I imagine you are at the very least curious to explore the Arc for your own benefit.

I promise you; you won't regret it. And I am always able to be contacted should you need my help. It would be my greatest privilege to be of service to your heart.

Remembering the way home to truly KNOW THYSELF as the human light being is the greatest journey you can take in your life. My greatest privilege has been showing you how this can be done.

Are you ready to give up on the old ideas of what you thought you were and discover what you were always meant to be?

Acknowledgements

I would like to thank the reader for spending their valuable time reading this book. I wrote it out of love, because I wanted to share the experiences through which I was fortunate enough to expand my consciousness. If you are in pain, as I was, physically or emotionally, and you want this ongoing suffering to stop, it may be time to go through and beyond your pain and stare into the happiness you were always intended to discover. I trust that this book gives you the opportunity to love your pain away, not just manage it or pay people to manage it for you.

I would also like to thank everyone I have interacted with in my life, for they have all helped me advance to a place of higher self-awareness. Without their teachings, I would not be who and what I am today. I thank them all for their inspirations of love.

My many experiences with the metaphysical realms have also been paramount in allowing me to discover my deepest truths, and have driven my desire to go inward, not outward, to transform my own life. It was here that I found my own light, and the reasons why I am alive today. I am therefore extremely grateful for the guidance I have received, and to those who have helped me access it. Sue Thompson (Channeler of Universal Wisdom, New Zealand), Ava Leonard (Body

Talk Practitioner, Australia), Paul Joseph (Spiritual Coach, Australia), Samantha Avery (Psychic Counsellor and Reiki Teacher, Australia), and Chensun Mills (Sacred Anatomy Energy Medicine Practitioner, USA) all gave me substantial access to inspirations and guidance beyond this physical world. All have amazing metaphysical abilities and levels of wisdom I was able to tap into to find my truths. All helped me to understand, and ultimately transcend, the pain I was mired within for over 50 years, and from there I was able to surrender to new beginnings.

Creating a book requires loving diligence and several people have helped me with this endeavour.

Zena Shapter, editor of all my books, has once again polished my manuscript to bring the pages I crafted to their full potentiality. The light that arises from within her and onto the pages that she edits is incredible.

Bill Shapter has turned my concept of the Arc into simple diagrams within this book. He is a master of the art of graphic design and has helped me with all my books.

Andrea Gussy has again helped me to construct and publish this book. This is a critical task I could not be without in my quest to write books from which readers can learn and find enjoyment. Wonderful friends with amazing talents like hers are such a blessing in one's life.

Julia Kuris designed the covers that grace this book. She is a wonderful woman with great artistic abilities. I am grateful that she helped to bring my words to light in such wonderful, colourful, and interesting ways.

As always, my five adult children have been a constant source of love and support for me as I have followed my dreams. Their never-ending acceptance of me, no matter what I do, has become a key foundation of the quest I undertook to find my truth and self-love. I love them very much.

About the Author

Mark Worthington discovered the concepts in this book because he is just like many of you – he had spent much of his life in pain and suffering. In his 50s, he finally decided to face his pain, to go through and beyond it, and improve the experiences of his sometimes-humbling life. Although he is far from perfect, this process led him to a higher self-awareness, and discoveries beyond his 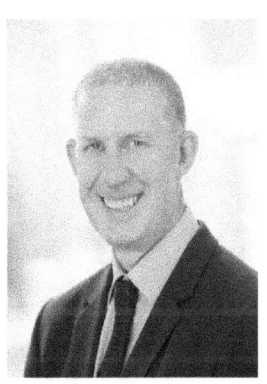 wildest dreams. This brought forth great truths and mysteries that were always within him, though he had never previously allowed himself to imagine them. By opening to his pain, Mark developed the Natural Arc of Human Transformation, and is now an avid proponent of the power of love and truth to transform people's lives and help them find happiness.

In 2022, Mark published *Where Your Happiness Hides*, depicting his deep and personal examination of human belief structures, and how they predetermine many experiences, limiting us and causing us much suffering.

In 2023, he published *Show Me the Harmony*, which explores just how conscious modern leaders can become. Mark has always possessed advanced leadership attributes that helped him to create organisations where people could feel united and able to express their true selves. In a modern world yearning for leaders who, through the application of real consciousness, truly know themselves and can lead their people effectively, this book is a must-read for the up-and-coming leaders of our future.

Mark is now passionate about assisting others with their journey to higher self-awareness. Should you desire his assistance, contact him through his website at: mark-worthington.com. He would love to hear from you!

www.ingramcontent.com/pod-product-compliance
Lightning Source LLC
Chambersburg PA
CBHW052133070526
44585CB00017B/1803